# The Lost Book

## of

# Nature's Healing Secrets

---

200+ Natural and Herbal Remedies for a Healthier, Chemical Pill-Free Life. Discover Ancient Wisdom and Modern Techniques for Holistic Healing.

**David Burke**

# Table of Content

# *Introduction*

In an era where the fast pace of modern life often leaves us disconnected from nature, there is a growing recognition of the importance of returning to our roots for health and wellness solutions. This book endeavors to bridge the gap between ancient wisdom and contemporary practices by offering a comprehensive guide to natural remedies that have stood the test of time. This book is designed to serve as a companion on the journey of seeking alternatives to synthetic medications, enhancing overall wellness, or simply becoming curious about the rich traditions of herbal medicine.

## *The Growing Trend Towards Holistic and Natural Healing*

In recent years, there has been a notable shift towards holistic and natural approaches to health and wellness. This trend is driven by a variety of factors, including increased awareness of the side effects associated with synthetic medications, a desire for more personalized and preventative healthcare, and a growing appreciation for the interconnectedness of mind, body, and spirit. Holistic healing is a therapeutic approach that prioritizes the treatment of the whole person, rather than merely addressing the symptoms, with the goal of restoring balance and promoting long-term well-being.

Natural remedies, which encompass herbal medicine, nutrition, and lifestyle practices, represent a gentler yet efficacious approach to health. These therapies work in harmony with the body's natural processes, supporting the immune system, reducing inflammation, and promoting overall vitality. As individuals become increasingly informed about their health options, the demand for natural and holistic solutions continues to grow.

## The Book's Comprehensive Nature and Historical Perspective

This book is designed to serve as a comprehensive reference for those interested in natural remedies. The book covers a wide range of topics, from the fundamental principles of herbal medicine to specific recipes for common ailments. By examining the historical context of herbal healing, the book offers a comprehensive account that bridges the gap between ancient traditions and contemporary practices.

An understanding of the historical context is essential for an appreciation of the evolution of herbal medicine and its continued relevance in the present. By examining the historical development of various remedies, readers can gain an appreciation for the depth of knowledge that has been passed down through generations. This comprehensive approach ensures that readers not only learn about the practical applications of natural remedies but also gain insight into the cultural and historical significance of these practices.

## The Relevance of Ancestral Wisdom in Modern Times

In our contemporary, technologically advanced society, there has been a resurgence of interest in the wisdom of our ancestors. Traditional practices, which were often grounded in a profound comprehension of the natural world, offer invaluable insights into the maintenance of health and the prevention of disease. Ancestral wisdom encompasses a holistic view of health that encompasses the physical, emotional, and spiritual aspects of well-being.

This book demonstrates how ancient practices can be adapted and integrated into modern lifestyles. For instance, the utilization of herbs for medicinal purposes has constituted a fundamental aspect of numerous cultures' healing traditions. These practices are not only efficacious but also sustainable, fostering a connection to nature that is often lacking in contemporary life.

Embracing ancestral wisdom can facilitate the attainment of equilibrium and concord in one's existence. This book encourages readers to explore these time-honored practices and discover how they can enhance their health and wellness in today's world. The book offers practical advice, detailed recipes, and a holistic approach to empower readers to take charge of their health using natural remedies that have been trusted for centuries.

## The Vital Essence of Natural Remedies

### The Importance of Natural Remedies in Contemporary Health Care

In the current landscape of healthcare, natural remedies are assuming an increasingly pivotal role. As the number of individuals seeking alternatives to conventional medicine continues to grow, the appeal of natural therapies is also on the rise. This shift is driven by a variety of factors, including the rising prevalence of chronic diseases, a greater awareness of the side effects associated with synthetic drugs, and a desire for more holistic and preventive healthcare approaches.

Natural remedies, which encompass herbs, essential oils, and dietary supplements, represent a more gentle approach to healing. They function in a complementary manner with the body's intrinsic processes, facilitating the restoration of equilibrium and the promotion of overall well-being. In contrast to many synthetic medications, which often target specific symptoms, natural remedies aim to address the root causes of illness. This holistic approach can result in more sustainable health outcomes, as it encourages the body's inherent capacity to heal itself.

Moreover, the integration of natural remedies into contemporary healthcare allows for more personalized treatment plans. The specific health needs of each individual are unique, and natural therapies can be tailored to meet these individual requirements. This personalized approach not only enhances the effectiveness of treatment but also empowers individuals to assume an active role in their health and wellness.

## *Advantages of Using Natural and Organic Methods Over Synthetic Medications*

A comparison of natural treatments with synthetic medications reveals several key advantages for the former. Firstly, natural remedies are often associated with fewer side effects than their synthetic counterparts. Synthetic drugs, while efficacious in numerous instances, can occasionally give rise to adverse reactions that result in the emergence of further health complications. In contrast, natural treatments are typically less intense and less prone to causing adverse effects, making them a safer choice for long-term use.

Another significant benefit of natural remedies is their holistic nature. In contrast to synthetic medications, which typically focus on alleviating specific symptoms, natural treatments consider the whole person, encompassing physical, emotional, and spiritual aspects of health. This comprehensive approach not only addresses the immediate health concern but also promotes overall well-being and balance.

Moreover, natural and organic methods frequently prioritize prevention and overall well-being, rather than merely treating disease. For instance, herbs and dietary supplements can be employed to fortify the immune system, diminish inflammation, and facilitate the body's intrinsic detoxification processes. By fostering a state of optimal health, natural remedies can help to prevent the onset of illness and improve the quality of life.

Furthermore, the use of natural remedies is in alignment with a growing interest in sustainable and eco-friendly living. A significant proportion of synthetic pharmaceuticals are derived from non-renewable resources, which can have a detrimental impact on the environment. Natural treatments, in particular those derived from organic sources, are more environmentally friendly and encourage a sustainable approach to healthcare.

Finally, natural remedies are often more accessible and cost-effective than synthetic medications. A multitude of herbs and natural supplements can be cultivated at home or procured from local markets, rendering them a viable option for those seeking cost-effective healthcare solutions.

The fundamental principle underlying the efficacy of natural remedies is their capacity to provide safe, holistic, and sustainable solutions.

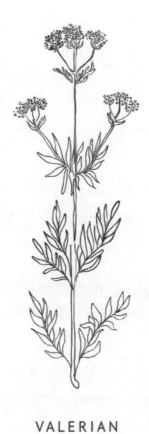

VALERIAN

# *Chapter 1: Holistic Nutrition*

Nutrition is the cornerstone of health, influencing all aspects of our well-being. In a world where processed foods and synthetic supplements are the dominant market forces, the importance of returning to natural, whole-food sources cannot be overstated. Holistic nutrition encompasses not only the nourishment of the body but also the consideration of the mind and spirit, thereby providing a comprehensive approach to wellness. This chapter explores the principles of holistic nutrition, with a particular focus on the potential of herbal healing, the concept of whole-person wellness, and the integration of ancestral wisdom into contemporary dietary practices.

## *The Essence of Herbal Healing: A Brief Overview*

The practice of herbal healing has been an integral part of human health for millennia. Long before the advent of modern medicine, our ancestors derived their medicinal needs from the natural world. Herbs were employed to treat a multitude of ailments, encompassing minor injuries such as cuts and bruises to more serious conditions such as infections and chronic diseases. This section offers a concise overview of the extensive history of herbal remedies, tracing their origins and evolution over time.

### *Historical Context of Herbal Remedies*

Herbs have been used for medicinal purposes since the dawn of time. The Egyptians, Chinese, Indians, Greeks, and Romans all developed sophisticated systems of herbal medicine. These early healers noticed how different plants affected people and wrote about their findings, creating a body of knowledge that has been passed down through the generations. For instance, the Ebers Papyrus, an ancient Egyptian medical document, lists hundreds of herbal remedies that were used to treat a variety of ailments.

In ancient China, herbal medicine was an essential part of Traditional Chinese Medicine (TCM), which placed a lot of emphasis on the balance of yin and yang and the flow of qi (vital energy) through the body. Likewise, Ayurveda, the traditional system of medicine in India, has relied on herbal remedies for thousands of years to promote health and longevity. The Greeks and Romans also made some truly amazing contributions to the field of herbal medicine! Hippocrates and Galen, for instance, laid the foundations for Western herbalism, which has been a driving force in the field ever since!

As herbal knowledge spread around the world, different cultures changed it to suit their needs. This is the basis of modern herbal medicine.

### Modern Resurgence of Interest in Natural Healing

People are interested in herbal and natural remedies again. This is due to many reasons. People are becoming more aware of the risks of synthetic drugs. Many people are looking for safer, natural treatments instead of conventional ones. Secondly, there is a broader movement towards holistic and integrative healthcare, which treats the whole person.

Furthermore, the Internet and the increased accessibility of information have also played a significant role in this revival. The advent of the internet has facilitated the dissemination of information about the benefits of herbal remedies, which has contributed to a greater acceptance and use of these natural therapies. Furthermore, the global wellness movement has underscored the significance of preventive care and the utilization of natural products to sustain health and forestall disease.

This renewed interest in herbal medicine is not merely a passing fad; it represents a profound shift towards embracing and integrating the insights of the past into contemporary healthcare practices.

### *The Synergy and Harmony in Herbal Medicine*

One of the fundamental principles of herbal medicine is the concept of synergy. In contrast to synthetic drugs, which frequently isolate a single active ingredient, herbal remedies employ the use of whole plants or combinations of plants. This holistic approach exploits the synergistic effects of the various compounds within the plant, which work in concert to enhance their therapeutic benefits.

For instance, an herb may contain compounds that reduce inflammation, while other components support the immune system or provide antioxidants. This synergy ensures that the body receives a balanced and comprehensive form of treatment. Furthermore, herbal medicine respects the body's natural processes, with the aim of supporting and enhancing the body's inherent ability to heal itself.

Moreover, herbal remedies are typically less invasive to the body than synthetic drugs. Furthermore, they are less likely to cause adverse effects or disrupt the body's natural equilibrium. By working in harmony with the body's systems, herbal medicine promotes overall wellness and helps to restore equilibrium.

The essence of herbal healing can be found in its historical roots, its modern resurgence, and its synergistic approach to health. By comprehending and espousing these tenets, we can harness the profound curative potential of herbs and integrate them into our holistic nutritional practices. This chapter will provide an introduction to the fundamental principles of herbal healing, laying the foundation for a more in-depth examination of holistic nutrition and wellness.

## Whole-Person Wellness

Holistic nutrition and wellness extend beyond the mere addressing of physical health. Rather, they encompass the entire spectrum of an individual's well-being, including mental, emotional, and spiritual aspects. The concept of whole-person wellness posits that true health is achieved by balancing and integrating all these components. This section explores the concept of whole-person wellness, emphasizing integrative approaches to health and the crucial mind-body connection in the healing process.

### Integrative Approaches to Health

Integrative health is an interdisciplinary approach that integrates various healing modalities to address the whole person, rather than merely treating the symptoms of a disease. It integrates conventional Western medicine with complementary and alternative therapies, thereby creating a personalized and holistic plan that is tailored to each individual's needs. The objective is to leverage the strengths of multiple disciplines in order to achieve optimal health and well-being.

Integrative approaches can include a combination of the following:

- *Conventional Medicine*: Traditional medical practices and treatments prescribed by healthcare professionals.

- *Herbal Medicine*: The use of plant-based remedies to support health and treat ailments.

- *Nutrition*: A focus on whole, nutrient-dense foods that nourish the body and support overall wellness.

- *Physical Therapies*: Practices such as yoga, tai chi, and chiropractic care that enhance physical health and mobility.

- *Mind-Body Techniques*: Approaches like meditation, mindfulness, and biofeedback that promote mental and emotional well-being.

- *Energy Therapies*: Modalities such as Reiki and acupuncture that work with the body's energy systems to facilitate healing.

The integration of these disparate modalities allows individuals to benefit from a comprehensive approach that addresses all facets of their health. This method acknowledges that no single therapeutic approach can address every health issue. It further recognizes that combining different therapeutic modalities can lead to more effective and sustainable outcomes.

## *Mind-Body Connection in Healing*

The mind-body connection is a fundamental principle in holistic health. It acknowledges that mental and emotional states significantly impact physical health, and vice versa. An understanding of this connection is of paramount importance for the attainment of whole-person wellness.

- *Mental Health and Physical Health*: It is becoming increasingly evident that stress, anxiety, and depression can manifest physically, resulting in a range of symptoms including headaches, digestive issues, and chronic pain. Conversely, the presence of physical illnesses can have a detrimental effect on mental and emotional well-being, thereby creating a vicious cycle that can be challenging to break. The recognition of this interplay allows for the implementation of more comprehensive treatment strategies that address both the mental and physical aspects of health.

- *Stress Reduction*: Chronic stress is a significant contributing factor to a multitude of health concerns, including cardiovascular disease, compromised immune function, and hormonal imbalances. Mind-body techniques, such as mindfulness meditation, deep breathing exercises, and yoga, have been demonstrated to significantly reduce stress levels, thereby promoting relaxation and improving overall health.

- **_Emotional Well-being_**: Emotions are of critical importance in the context of physical health. The practice of journaling, therapy, and engaging in creative activities can assist in the processing of emotions and the reduction of their negative impact on the body. It has been demonstrated that positive emotions, such as joy and gratitude, can enhance immune function and promote healing.

- **_Holistic Healing Practices_**: Integrative therapies frequently emphasise the significance of the mind-body connection. For example, acupuncture addresses not only physical symptoms but also aims to balance the body's energy flow, which can positively influence mental health. Similarly, herbal remedies may be selected not only for their physical benefits but also for their capacity to support emotional and mental well-being.

- **_Lifestyle Changes_**: The incorporation of mind-body practices into daily routines has been demonstrated to result in long-term enhancements in health and well-being. Regular physical activity, adequate sleep, a balanced diet, and stress management techniques all contribute to a harmonious balance between mind and body.

The concept of whole-person wellness is predicated on the recognition and nurturing of the interconnectedness of our physical, mental, and emotional health. By adopting integrative approaches and honoring the mind-body connection, individuals can achieve a more balanced, healthy, and fulfilling life. This section is designed to provide insights and practical advice on how to integrate these principles into everyday life, thereby fostering a deeper understanding and appreciation of holistic wellness.

# Ancestral Wisdom and Cultural Tradition

A comprehensive examination of the field of holistic nutrition would be incomplete without an acknowledgment of the profound historical and cultural influences that have shaped the use of herbs throughout history. Ancestral wisdom and cultural heritage have profoundly influenced how we understand and utilize herbal remedies in the present day. This section examines the traditional uses of herbs across various cultures and the role of cultural heritage in modern herbal practices.

## Traditional Uses of Herbs Across Different Cultures

Herbs have constituted a fundamental component of traditional medicine in a multitude of cultures across the globe. Each culture has developed its own distinctive system of herbal medicine, shaped by its unique environment, spiritual beliefs, and understanding of health and disease.

- *Traditional Chinese Medicine (TCM)*: TCM has employed the use of herbs for millennia, with a focus on the balancing of the body's energy, or qi. Chinese herbal medicine encompasses a comprehensive pharmacopeia of remedies designed to harmonize yin and yang, addressing both the root causes and symptoms of illness.

- *Ayurveda*: The ancient Indian system of medicine, Ayurveda, places significant emphasis on the balance of the body, mind, and spirit. Ayurvedic practitioners utilize herbs to regulate the three doshas (Vata, Pitta, and Kapha) and enhance overall health. The most commonly utilized Ayurvedic herbs include turmeric, ashwagandha, and holy basil.

- **_Native American Medicine_**: The indigenous tribes of North America have a longstanding tradition of herbal medicine, with a rich history of utilising local flora for therapeutic purposes. Herbs such as echinacea, sage, and yarrow have been utilized for their medicinal properties, often in conjunction with spiritual practices and rituals.

- **_European Herbal Medicine_**: In Europe, the history of herbal medicine is long and rich, with roots extending back to ancient Greece and Rome. The contributions of figures such as Hippocrates and Galen laid the foundations for Western herbalism, which continued to evolve throughout the Middle Ages and Renaissance. Herbs such as chamomile, nettle, and elderberry have constituted a significant component of European herbal practices.

- **_African Traditional Medicine_**: African cultures have developed a diverse array of herbal remedies that are tailored to the continent's varied ecosystems. In traditional African medicine, practitioners known as sangomas employ a variety of plant-based remedies, including rooibos, aloe, and devil's claw, which they utilize for their therapeutic benefits.

- **_Latin American Herbal Traditions_**: Latin American herbal practices frequently integrate indigenous knowledge with influences from Spanish and African cultures. Herbs such as maca, uña de gato, and chanca piedra are frequently employed for their purported health benefits.

## The Role of Cultural Heritage in Modern Herbal Practices

Cultural heritage continues to be a significant factor in contemporary herbal practices. Many contemporary herbalists draw upon the accumulated wisdom of their forebears, integrating traditional knowledge with contemporary scientific understanding. This integration of traditional and contemporary knowledge provides a more comprehensive and effective approach to herbal medicine.

- *Preservation of Knowledge*: Cultural heritage plays a pivotal role in the preservation of extensive knowledge pertaining to herbal medicine. The transmission of traditional practices from one generation to the next ensures the perpetuation of valuable information about plant properties and uses.

- *Inspiration for Innovation*: Modern herbalists frequently draw upon traditional practices as a source of inspiration, adapting ancient remedies to address contemporary health challenges. This approach enables the development of novel, cutting-edge treatments that are firmly rooted in time-honored wisdom.

- *Cultural Identity and Healing*: For a significant proportion of the population, the use of herbs represents a means of establishing a connection with their cultural identity and heritage. This connection can facilitate the healing process by providing a sense of belonging and continuity.

- *Ethical and Sustainable Practices*: Cultural traditions place a premium on the sustainable and respectful use of natural resources. By adhering to these tenets, contemporary herbalists can ensure that their practices are environmentally responsible and ethically sound.

- ***Integration into Modern Healthcare***: Cultural heritage plays a role in the integration of herbal medicine into mainstream healthcare. As the medical community increasingly recognizes the value of holistic approaches, traditional herbal practices are being integrated into conventional treatments.

As we progress, Chapter 2 will provide a more profound examination of the core principles of herbal medicine. The practical aspects of Nature's Pharmacy will be explored, including an examination of the benefits and uses of specific herbs, an investigation of plant properties, and an investigation of the methods for identifying and sourcing quality herbs. This chapter will provide the foundational knowledge necessary to effectively harness the power of medicinal plants, offering a detailed guide to incorporating these natural remedies into one's daily life.

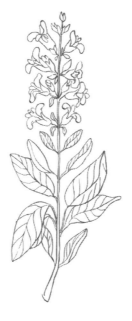

SAGE

# Chapter 2: Nature's Pharmacy

In the field of natural healing, herbs are among the most efficacious agents available. Herbs form the foundation of traditional medical systems worldwide and continue to be a vital component of contemporary holistic health practices. This chapter will provide an overview of the essential principles of herbal medicine, offering practical insights into the benefits and uses of various herbs. This chapter will examine the properties and applications of medicinal plants, exploring their key characteristics and providing guidance on how to identify and source high-quality herbs. By the conclusion of this chapter, the reader will have acquired the requisite knowledge to integrate these efficacious plants into their personal wellness regimen with confidence.

## Benefits and Uses of Herbs

Herbs are renowned for their ability to support and enhance health in numerous ways. From enhancing the immune system to alleviating stress, the benefits of these natural remedies are extensive. In order to fully exploit the potential of herbs, it is essential to gain an understanding of their distinctive properties and applications.

### Understanding Plant Properties and Their Applications

Medicinal plants contain a diverse array of bioactive compounds that contribute to their healing properties. These compounds can exert a variety of effects on the body, including anti-inflammatory, antimicrobial, antioxidant, and adaptogenic actions. The following paragraphs will present a selection of the most important properties of medicinal plants and their applications:

- ***Anti-inflammatory***: Herbs such as turmeric and ginger contain bioactive compounds, namely curcumin and gingerol, respectively, which have anti-inflammatory properties and are commonly employed in the management of conditions such as arthritis and muscle pain.

- ***Antimicrobial***: Garlic and oregano possess intrinsic antimicrobial properties, rendering them efficacious against a spectrum of bacteria, viruses, and fungi. These herbs have the potential to be utilized as a preventative and therapeutic agent in the treatment of infections.

- ***Antioxidant***: Herbs such as green tea and rosemary are rich in antioxidants, which help to protect the body from oxidative stress and free radical damage. This property is beneficial for the prevention of chronic diseases and the promotion of overall health.

- ***Adaptogenic***: Adaptogenic herbs, such as ashwagandha and rhodiola, assist the body in adapting to stress and maintaining homeostasis. These herbs are frequently employed to enhance energy, reduce fatigue, and improve resilience to stress.

- ***Digestive***: Herbs such as peppermint and fennel have been demonstrated to support digestive health by alleviating symptoms associated with indigestion, bloating, and flatulence. These herbs can be employed to enhance digestive health and to alleviate gastrointestinal discomfort.

## Key Characteristics of Medicinal Plants

The identification of medicinal herbs necessitates the recognition of their distinctive characteristics. The following characteristics should be observed:

- **Leaf Shape and Arrangement**: The shape, size, and arrangement of leaves can be employed to identify a plant. For instance, peppermint exhibits oval, serrated leaves that grow in opposition to each other along the stem.

- **Flowers**: The color, shape, and arrangement of flowers are also important identifiers. For example, chamomile is distinguished by its small, white, daisy-like flowers with a yellow center.

- **Aroma**: A number of medicinal herbs possess a distinctive scent. For example, lavender is readily identifiable by its soothing, floral aroma.

- **Roots and Stems**: The structure and color of roots and stems can serve as distinguishing features. Echinacea, for instance, is characterised by a fibrous root system and a sturdy, hairy stem.

- **Seeds and Fruit**: The appearance of seeds and fruits can be utilized as a means of identification. The seeds of milk thistle exhibit a distinctive black and white coloration, which is attributed to their hepatoprotective properties.


## Identifying and Sourcing Quality Herbs

In order to guarantee the efficacy and security of herbal remedies, it is of the utmost importance to identify and procure high-quality herbs. The following guidelines are provided for your consideration:

- **Sourcing**: It is advisable to purchase herbs from suppliers who prioritize quality and sustainability. It is advisable to select herbs that have been certified as organic, as this ensures that they are free from pesticides and other harmful chemicals.

- **Harvesting**: Those who harvest their own herbs are encouraged to do so in a responsible manner. It is advisable to harvest at the optimal time, when the plant's medicinal properties are at their peak. It is advisable to avoid harvesting the plant in excess, in order to ensure the continued health of the population.

- **Appearance**: It is expected that high-quality dried herbs will retain their natural color and have a vibrant appearance. It is advisable to avoid herbs that exhibit signs of deterioration, such as discoloration or mold growth.

- **Aroma**: Fresh and dried herbs should exhibit a robust, distinctive aroma. A lack of scent may be indicative of the herbs being old or of poor quality.

- **Storage**: It is recommended that herbs be stored in airtight containers away from light, heat, and moisture in order to preserve their potency. Proper storage techniques help to maintain the beneficial properties of herbs over time.

By comprehending the characteristics and identifying attributes of medicinal plants, as well as procuring them in an ethical manner, one can optimally leverage the potential of Nature's Pharmacy. The subsequent sections of this chapter will provide a more detailed examination of specific herbs, their benefits, and practical applications. This will equip the reader with the knowledge necessary to effectively utilize these natural remedies in their daily lives.

## The Doctrine's Historical Background

An understanding of the historical context of herbal medicine not only enhances our appreciation of these natural remedies but also provides practical insights into their effective use. The doctrine of signatures, a historical concept, played a significant role in the development of herbal medicine. This doctrine posits that the physical characteristics of plants, including their shape, color, and habitat, are indicative of their medicinal properties. Although not empirically substantiated, this ancient wisdom has influenced the selection and combination of herbs throughout history.

## Practical Applications in Choosing and Combining Herbs

The selection and combination of herbs necessitates both knowledge and intuition, frequently informed by traditional practices and contemporary understanding. The following section outlines a number of practical methods for the effective selection and combination of herbs for a variety of applications.

## Understanding the Doctrine of Signatures

The doctrine of signatures is based on the idea that plants resemble the parts of the body or the ailments they can help treat. For instance:

- **Lungwort (Pulmonaria)**: The leaves of lungwort exhibit a pattern that resembles lung tissue, and it has been traditionally employed in the treatment of respiratory conditions.

- **Walnut**: The shape of a walnut is reminiscent of the human brain, and research has demonstrated that walnuts are beneficial for brain health due to their high omega-3 fatty acid content.

- **Eyebright (Euphrasia)**: The flowers of the plant Euphrasia, commonly known as eyebright, bear a striking resemblance to the human eye. For centuries, they have been employed in the treatment of eye infections and as a means of improving vision.

Although modern science does not fully corroborate these associations, they offer a fascinating insight into the historical approaches to herbal medicine.

## Combining Herbs for Synergistic Effects

The combination of herbs can enhance their efficacy through the phenomenon of synergy, whereby the combined action of multiple herbs is greater than the sum of their individual effects. The following principles should be considered when combining herbs effectively:

- **Complementary Actions**: It is advisable to combine herbs that have complementary actions. For instance, the combination of anti-inflammatory herbs (such as turmeric) with immune-boosting herbs (such as echinacea) can provide comprehensive support for the body's healing processes.

- **Balancing Energies**: In traditional systems such as Ayurveda and Traditional Chinese Medicine (TCM), herbs are frequently combined in order to achieve a balance between their energetic properties, which may include effects such as warming and cooling. This ensures that the blend is harmonized and suitable for the individual's constitution.

- **Supporting Functions**: It is recommended that herbs be combined that support different functions of the body. For example, a digestive tonic might include herbs that stimulate digestion (such as ginger), soothe the digestive tract (such as licorice), and reduce inflammation (such as chamomile).

- **Enhancing Absorption**: It has been demonstrated that certain herbs facilitate the absorption of other herbs. For instance, black pepper (piperine) is frequently incorporated into turmeric formulations with the objective of enhancing the bioavailability of curcumin, the active compound in turmeric.

- **Formulation Ratios**: It is of paramount importance to pay close attention to the ratios when combining herbs. The primary herb, which is the one with the primary therapeutic action, is typically used in the highest amount, while the supportive herbs are used in smaller quantities to enhance the primary herb's effects.

## Practical Tips for Choosing Herbs

- **Identify the Health Concern**: It is essential to delineate the specific health issue that is to be addressed. This process facilitates the identification of herbs with specific actions that are pertinent to the condition in question.

- **Research and Knowledge**: It is recommended that reliable sources be utilized in order to conduct research pertaining to the properties and applications of various herbs. It is of the utmost importance to gain an understanding of the actions, contraindications, and interactions of these substances.

- **Quality Matters**: It is advisable to select herbs of the highest quality. It is advisable to source herbs from reputable suppliers and to consider organic options in order to ensure that the herbs are free from contaminants.

- **Experiment and Adjust**: The practice of herbal medicine frequently entails some degree of experimentation. It is advisable to commence with a relatively low dose and observe the subsequent physiological response. It is necessary to adjust the combination and dosage as required.

- **Consultation**: Should you be uncertain, it is advisable to seek the counsel of a duly qualified herbalist or healthcare professional. Such professionals can provide personalized advice and ensure that the herbal regimen is safe and effective.

By integrating historical insights with practical applications, it is possible to fully exploit the potential of herbal remedies. An understanding of the doctrine of signatures and the ability to effectively combine herbs can facilitate the development of more effective and holistic approaches to health and wellness.

# Chapter 3: Developing an Intimate Relationship with Plants

The development of a profound and personal connection with plants extends beyond the comprehension of their physical characteristics and therapeutic applications. It entails the recognition and exploitation of their energetic properties, the appreciation of the role of taste in herbal medicine, and the valuation of the sensory experiences they provide. This chapter examines these aspects and instructs readers on how to establish a more profound connection with herbs, thereby enabling them to fully exploit their healing potential.

## The Energetic Properties of Herbs

Herbs possess distinctive energetic properties that affect their impact on the body and mind. These properties can be employed to restore equilibrium and facilitate healing.

### How to Harness These Properties for Healing

- *Identifying Energetic Qualities*: Herbs can be classified according to their energetic properties, such as warming, cooling, drying, or humidifying. For example:
  - Warming Herbs: Ginger, cinnamon, and garlic. These herbs have been demonstrated to stimulate circulation and are

therefore useful in the treatment of conditions that are characterised by cold or stagnation.

- o Cooling Herbs: Peppermint, chamomile, and aloe vera. These herbs soothe inflammation and are beneficial for hot, irritated conditions.

- o Drying Herbs: Sage, thyme, and horsetail. These products are beneficial in damp conditions, such as mucus buildup or excessive sweating.

- o Moistening Herbs: Marshmallow root, slippery elm, and licorice. These herbs have the capacity to hydrate tissues and are therefore beneficial in the treatment of dry, irritated conditions.

- *Matching Herbs to Conditions*: It is advisable to select herbs whose energetic properties correspond to the condition being treated. For instance, the use of cooling herbs may be employed to treat fever or inflammation, whereas warming herbs may be employed to stimulate a sluggish digestive system.

- *Personal Constitution*: It is important to consider the individual's constitution, which encompasses their tendency to feel cold or hot, dry or moist. This personalized approach ensures that the herbs chosen will harmonize with the person's natural state and promote balance.

- *Seasonal Adjustments*: It is advisable to align one's herbal choices with the seasons. In order to counteract the effects of the cold in the winter and the heat in the summer, it is advisable to utilise warming herbs and cooling herbs, respectively.

## Understanding the Role of Taste in Herbal Medicine

The perception of taste plays a pivotal role in herbal medicine, as it can provide insights into an herb's energetic properties and therapeutic actions. In the context of herbal medicine, the five primary tastes are bitter, sweet, sour, salty, and pungent. Each taste is associated with specific effects.

- *Bitter*: It stimulates digestion, detoxifies the body, and supports liver function. Examples of such herbs include dandelion root and gentian.

- *Sweet*: This substance nourishes, soothes, and builds strength. Examples of such herbs include licorice and astragalus.

- *Sour*: These properties are collectively referred to as astringent, preservative, and stabilizing. Examples of such plants include lemon balm and hawthorn.

- *Salty*: It has the capacity to soften, dissolve, and detoxify. Examples of such substances include kelp and nettle.

- *Pungent*: It stimulates circulation and clears congestion. Examples of such substances include ginger and cayenne.

The use of taste as a guide to the selection of herbs facilitates the creation of balanced formulas that support overall health.

## Sensory Experiences and Their Healing Implications

- The experience of herbs extends beyond the sense of taste, encompassing the senses of sight, smell, and touch. These sensory interactions have the potential to enhance the healing process.

- *Aroma*: The olfactory perception of herbs has been demonstrated to exert a profound influence on mood and emotional well-being. Aromatic herbs such as lavender, rosemary, and peppermint can be employed in aromatherapy to reduce stress and promote relaxation.

- *Visual Appeal*: The chromatic and morphological diversity of herbs can be perceived as a source of inspiration and provide a visual representation of their properties. For instance, the bright yellow of calendula is indicative of its sunny, uplifting qualities.

- *Touch*: The act of handling herbs, whether through gardening or the preparation of remedies, creates a tangible connection that can be both grounding and therapeutic. The act of working with plants fosters a deeper appreciation and connection.

- *Holistic Engagement*: The engagement of all the senses in herbal practices has been demonstrated to promote mindfulness and enhance the overall healing experience. The preparation and utilization of herbal remedies can be regarded as a meditative and intentional practice.

An intimate relationship with plants can facilitate the effective harnessing of their energetic properties, the appreciation of the therapeutic role of taste, and the enrichment of the healing journey through sensory experiences.

The following chapter will present a compendium of 300 herbal recipes, each designed to address a specific ailment. The reader will learn how to combine herbs for enhanced efficacy, create synergistic blends, and prepare detailed recipes for specific health issues. With detailed instructions for preparation and use, Chapter 4 will enable readers to integrate these efficacious remedies into their daily health routines, providing natural solutions for vibrant well-being.

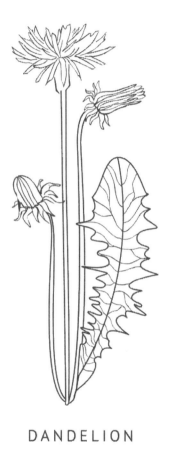

DANDELION

# Chapter 4: 180 Herbal Recipes

Herbs have been utilized for millennia to address a multitude of health concerns. This chapter presents 180 meticulously selected herbal recipes, designed to address common ailments, enhance overall wellness, and support specific health needs. The combination of herbs to maximize their effectiveness, the creation of synergistic blends, and the provision of detailed preparation instructions are the means by which this chapter aims to equip the reader with practical tools to harness the healing power of nature.

## Recipes for Common Ailments

Herbal remedies offer a natural and effective solution for a multitude of common health issues. By understanding how to combine herbs for enhanced efficacy and creating synergistic blends, it is possible to tailor remedies to address specific conditions.

### Combining Herbs for Enhanced Efficacy

The combination of herbs can result in a more potent remedy by leveraging the complementary actions of different plants. The following paragraphs will present some key principles and examples.

## 1. Immune Boosting Blend:

Ingredients: Echinacea, elderberry, astragalus, and ginger.

Benefits: Echinacea and elderberry have been demonstrated to support immune function, while astragalus has been shown to strengthen overall vitality. Ginger, meanwhile, has been found to possess anti-inflammatory and warming properties.

Recipe: A combination of equal parts of dried echinacea root, elderberries, and astragalus root should be prepared. At this juncture, it is advisable to incorporate a smaller quantity of dried ginger root. One tablespoon of the aforementioned blend should be simmered in two cups of water for approximately fifteen minutes. The resulting liquid should be strained and consumed in quantities of one to two cups per day during the period of increased susceptibility to colds and flu.

## 2. Digestive Aid Tea:

Ingredients: Peppermint, fennel, and chamomile.

Benefits: Peppermint has been demonstrated to have a soothing effect on the digestive tract, fennel has been shown to relieve gas and bloating, and chamomile has been found to calm and support digestion.

Recipe: A suitable proportion of the ingredients is to be combined, namely equal parts of dried peppermint leaves, fennel seeds, and chamomile flowers. One teaspoon of the blend should be steeped in one cup of hot water for ten minutes. The resulting infusion should be strained and consumed after meals.

### 3. Stress Relief Blend:

Ingredients: Ashwagandha, holy basil, and lemon balm.

Benefits: Ashwagandha has been demonstrated to reduce stress and anxiety, holy basil has been shown to act as an adaptogen, thereby maintaining equilibrium within the body, and lemon balm has been found to promote relaxation.

Recipe: Combine equal parts of dried ashwagandha root, holy basil leaves, and lemon balm leaves. Steep 1 teaspoon of the blend in 1 cup of hot water for 15 minutes. Strain and drink 1-2 times daily.

### 4. Anti-Inflammatory Tea:

Ingredients: Turmeric, ginger, and cinnamon.

Benefits: Turmeric and ginger reduce inflammation, and cinnamon adds antioxidant properties.

Recipe: The ingredients should be combined in a ratio of two parts turmeric root, one part ginger root, and one part cinnamon bark. One teaspoon of the aforementioned blend should be simmered in one cup of water for a period of ten minutes. The mixture should be strained and consumed twice daily.

### 5. Energy Boosting Tea:

Ingredients: Ginseng, green tea, and licorice root.

Benefits: Ginseng has been demonstrated to enhance energy levels, green tea provides a mild stimulant effect, and antioxidants, such as those found in licorice root, have been shown to support adrenal health.

Recipe: Combine equal parts of dried ginseng root, green tea leaves, and licorice root. Steep 1 teaspoon of the blend in 1 cup of hot water for 5 minutes. Strain and drink in the morning.

## 6. Skin Health Blend:

Ingredients: Calendula, burdock root, and nettle.

Benefits: Calendula is known to promote skin healing, burdock root is a detoxifying agent, and nettle provides essential nutrients.

Recipe: Combine equal parts of dried calendula flowers, burdock root, and nettle leaves. One teaspoon of the blend should be steeped in one cup of hot water for ten minutes. The solution should be strained and consumed on a daily basis.

## 7. Anti-Anxiety Blend:

Ingredients: Lavender, passionflower, and skullcap.

Benefits: Lavender and passionflower reduce anxiety, and skullcap supports the nervous system.

Recipe: A combination of equal parts of dried lavender flowers, passionflower leaves, and skullcap should be prepared. Steep 1 teaspoon of the blend in 1 cup of hot water for 15 minutes. Strain and drink as needed.

### 8. Detox Tea:

Ingredients: Dandelion root, milk thistle, and burdock root.

Benefits: Dandelion root and milk thistle have been demonstrated to support liver detoxification, while burdock root has been shown to facilitate overall cleansing.

Recipe: Combine equal parts of dried dandelion root, milk thistle seeds, and burdock root. One tablespoon of the blend should be simmered in two cups of water for fifteen minutes. The resulting liquid should be strained and consumed on a daily basis.

### 9. Respiratory Support Tea:

Ingredients: Mullein, thyme, and elecampane.

Benefits: Mullein soothes the respiratory tract, thyme acts as an antimicrobial, and elecampane supports lung health.

Recipe: A suitable proportion of the ingredients is to be combined, namely equal parts of dried mullein leaves, thyme, and elecampane root. One teaspoon of the blend should be steeped in one cup of hot water for ten minutes. The solution should be strained and consumed twice daily.

### 10. Menstrual Relief Blend:

Ingredients: Red raspberry leaf, cramp bark, and ginger.

Benefits: Red raspberry leaf has been demonstrated to tone the uterus, cramp bark has been shown to relieve menstrual cramps, and ginger has been found to reduce inflammation.

Recipe: Combine equal parts of dried red raspberry leaf, cramp bark, and ginger root. One teaspoon of the blend should be steeped in one cup of hot water for ten minutes. The solution should then be strained and consumed as required.

## 11. Memory and Focus Tea:

Ingredients: Ginkgo biloba, rosemary, and gotu kola.

Benefits: Ginkgo biloba has been demonstrated to improve cerebral circulation, rosemary has been shown to enhance cognitive function, and gotu kola has been found to support mental clarity.

Recipe: A combination of equal parts of dried ginkgo biloba leaves, rosemary, and gotu kola should be prepared. Steep 1 teaspoon of the blend in 1 cup of hot water for 10 minutes. Strain and drink once daily.

## 12. Anti-Depression Blend:

Ingredients: St. John's wort, lemon balm, and saffron.

Benefits: St. John's wort helps elevate mood, lemon balm calms the mind, and saffron boosts serotonin levels.

Recipe: Combine equal parts of dried St. John's wort, lemon balm, and saffron. One teaspoon of the blend should be steeped in one cup of hot water for ten minutes. The mixture should be strained and consumed on an as-needed basis.

### 13. Anti-Nausea Tea:

Ingredients: Ginger, peppermint, and fennel.

Benefits: Ginger and peppermint relieve nausea, and fennel soothes the digestive tract.

Recipe: A combination of equal parts of dried ginger root, peppermint leaves, and fennel seeds should be prepared. Steep 1 teaspoon of the blend in 1 cup of hot water for 10 minutes. Strain and drink as needed.


### 14. Arthritis Relief Blend:

Ingredients: Turmeric, devil's claw, and willow bark.

Benefits: The anti-inflammatory properties of turmeric and devil's claw, along with the analgesic effects of willow bark, have been well-documented in scientific literature.

Recipe: Combine equal parts of dried turmeric root, devil's claw, and willow bark. One teaspoon of the blend should be simmered in one cup of water for ten minutes. The solution should be strained and consumed twice daily.


### 15. Cold and Flu Tea:

Ingredients: Elderflower, yarrow, and peppermint.

Benefits: Elderflower has been demonstrated to enhance the immune system, while yarrow has been shown to reduce fever, and peppermint has been found to alleviate respiratory symptoms.

Recipe: A suitable proportion of the dried flowers of the elderflower, yarrow, and peppermint is to be combined. One teaspoon of the blend should be steeped in one cup of hot water for ten minutes. The solution should be strained and consumed two to three times daily during the course of the illness.

### 16. Joint Health Blend:

Ingredients: Boswellia, turmeric, and ginger.

Benefits: The botanical compounds boswellia and turmeric have been demonstrated to possess anti-inflammatory properties, while the spice ginger has been shown to enhance circulation and relieve pain.

Recipe: Combine equal parts of dried boswellia, turmeric, and ginger root. One teaspoon of the blend should be simmered in one cup of water for ten minutes. The solution should be strained and consumed on a daily basis.

### 17. Heart Health Tea:

Ingredients: Hawthorn, motherwort, and hibiscus.

Benefits: Hawthorn supports heart function, motherwort calms the heart, and hibiscus lowers blood pressure.

Recipe: A combination of equal parts of dried hawthorn berries, motherwort, and hibiscus flowers should be prepared. Steep 1 teaspoon of the blend in 1 cup of hot water for 10 minutes. Strain and drink once daily.

### 18. Diabetes Support Blend:

Ingredients: Cinnamon, fenugreek, and bilberry.

Benefits: Cinnamon has been demonstrated to regulate blood sugar, fenugreek has been shown to improve insulin sensitivity, and bilberry has been found to support eye health.

Recipe: Combine equal parts of dried cinnamon bark, fenugreek seeds, and bilberry leaves. Steep 1 teaspoon of the blend in 1 cup of hot water for 10 minutes. Strain and drink twice daily.

### 19. Kidney Support Tea:

Ingredients: Nettle, dandelion leaf, and corn silk.

Benefits: Nettle supports kidney function, dandelion leaf acts as a diuretic, and corn silk soothes the urinary tract.

Recipe: Combine equal parts of dried nettle leaves, dandelion leaf, and corn silk. One teaspoon of the blend should be steeped in one cup of hot water for ten minutes. The solution should be strained and consumed twice daily.

### 20. Thyroid Support Blend:

Ingredients: Ashwagandha, bladderwrack, and licorice root.

Benefits: Ashwagandha supports thyroid function, bladderwrack provides iodine, and licorice root balances hormones.

Recipe: A combination of equal parts of dried ashwagandha root, bladderwrack, and licorice root should be prepared. Steep 1 teaspoon of the blend in 1 cup of hot water for 10 minutes. Strain and drink once daily.

### 21. Liver Detox Tea:

Ingredients: Milk thistle, dandelion root, and turmeric.

Benefits: Milk thistle and dandelion root detoxify the liver, and turmeric reduces inflammation.

Recipe: Combine equal parts of dried milk thistle seeds, dandelion root, and turmeric root. One teaspoon of the blend should be simmered in one cup of water for ten minutes. The solution should be strained and consumed on a daily basis.

## 22. Circulation Boosting Blend:

Ingredients: Ginkgo biloba, cayenne, and ginger.

Benefits: Ginkgo biloba has been demonstrated to improve circulation, while cayenne has been shown to stimulate blood flow. Ginger has also been found to enhance overall circulation.

Recipe: Combine equal parts of dried ginkgo biloba leaves, cayenne pepper, and ginger root. Steep 1 teaspoon of the blend in 1 cup of hot water for 10 minutes. Strain and drink once daily.

## 23. Muscle Relaxation Tea:

Ingredients: Valerian, chamomile, and lavender.

Benefits: Valerian relaxes muscles, chamomile soothes, and lavender calms the mind.

Recipe: A suitable ratio for combining the dried valerian root, chamomile flowers, and lavender flowers is one part of each. One teaspoon of the blend should be steeped in one cup of hot water for ten minutes. The solution should then be strained and consumed as required.

## 24. Menopause Relief Blend:

Ingredients: Black cohosh, red clover, and sage.

Benefits: Black cohosh reduces hot flashes, red clover balances hormones, and sage reduces sweating.

Recipe: Combine equal parts of dried black cohosh, red clover, and sage. Steep 1 teaspoon of the blend in 1 cup of hot water for 10 minutes. Strain and drink twice daily.


## 25. Weight Loss Support Tea:

Ingredients: Green tea, dandelion root, and cinnamon.

Benefits: Green tea boosts metabolism, dandelion root acts as a diuretic, and cinnamon helps regulate blood sugar.

Recipe: Combine equal parts of dried green tea leaves, dandelion root, and cinnamon bark. One teaspoon of the blend should be steeped in one cup of hot water for a period of five minutes. The solution should be strained and consumed on a daily basis.


## 26. Bone Health Blend:

Ingredients: Horsetail, nettle, and oat straw.

Benefits: Horsetail is a source of silica, nettle provides minerals, and oat straw supports bone density.

Recipe: Combine equal parts of dried horsetail, nettle, and oat straw. Steep 1 teaspoon of the blend in 1 cup of hot water for 10 minutes. Strain and drink once daily.

## 27. Eye Health Tea:

Ingredients: Bilberry, eyebright, and goji berry.

Benefits: Bilberry supports eye health, eyebright soothes the eyes, and goji berry provides antioxidants.

Recipe: A suitable proportion of the ingredients is to be combined, namely equal parts of dried bilberry leaves, eyebright, and goji berries. One teaspoon of the blend should be steeped in one cup of hot water for ten minutes. The mixture should be strained and consumed on an as-needed basis.


## 28. Immune System Booster:

Ingredients: Reishi mushroom, astragalus, and elderberry.

Benefits: Reishi mushroom enhances immune function, astragalus boosts overall vitality, and elderberry fights infections.

Recipe: A combination of equal parts of dried reishi mushroom, astragalus root, and elderberries should be prepared. Simmer 1 tablespoon of the blend in 2 cups of water for 15 minutes. Strain and drink 1-2 cups daily.


## 29. Blood Pressure Lowering Tea:

Ingredients: Hibiscus, hawthorn, and garlic.

Benefits: Hibiscus lowers blood pressure, hawthorn supports heart health, and garlic improves circulation.

Recipe: Combine equal parts of dried hibiscus flowers, hawthorn berries, and garlic. One teaspoon of the blend should be steeped in one cup of hot water for ten minutes. The solution should be strained and consumed on a daily basis.

## 30. Digestive Health Blend:

Ingredients: Dandelion root, burdock root, and ginger.

Benefits: Dandelion root has been demonstrated to support digestive processes, burdock root has been shown to facilitate detoxification, and ginger has been found to possess anti-inflammatory properties.

Recipe: Combine equal parts of dried dandelion root, burdock root, and ginger root. Simmer 1 teaspoon of the blend in 1 cup of water for 10 minutes. Strain and drink twice daily.

## 31. Allergy Relief Tea:

Ingredients: Nettle, peppermint, and eyebright.

Benefits: Nettle reduces histamine response, peppermint clears sinuses, and eyebright soothes the eyes.

Recipe: A suitable proportion of the ingredients is to be combined, namely equal parts of dried nettle leaves, peppermint leaves, and eyebright. One teaspoon of the aforementioned blend should be steeped in one cup of boiling water for a period of ten minutes. The solution should then be strained and consumed as needed.

## 32. Endurance Enhancing Blend:

Ingredients: Rhodiola, ginseng, and maca.

Benefits: Rhodiola improves stamina, ginseng boosts energy, and maca enhances physical performance.

Recipe: A combination of equal parts of dried rhodiola root, ginseng root, and maca root should be prepared. Steep 1 teaspoon of the blend in 1 cup of hot water for 10 minutes. Strain and drink once daily.

### 33. Heartburn Relief Tea:

Ingredients: Marshmallow root, licorice root, and slippery elm.

Benefits: Marshmallow root soothes the digestive tract, licorice root heals, and slippery elm coats the stomach lining.

Recipe: Combine equal parts of dried marshmallow root, licorice root, and slippery elm. One teaspoon of the blend should be steeped in one cup of hot water for ten minutes. The solution should then be strained and consumed as required.

### 34. Liver Health Blend:

Ingredients: Milk thistle, artichoke leaf, and dandelion root.

Benefits: The consumption of milk thistle has been demonstrated to facilitate the detoxification of the liver, while artichoke leaf and dandelion root have been shown to support liver function and promote detoxification, respectively.

Recipe: Combine equal parts of dried milk thistle seeds, artichoke leaf, and dandelion root. Simmer 1 teaspoon of the blend in 1 cup of water for 10 minutes. Strain and drink once daily.

## 35. Anxiety Relief Tea:

Ingredients: Lemon balm, valerian, and chamomile.

Benefits: Lemon balm calms the mind, valerian reduces anxiety, and chamomile promotes relaxation.

Recipe: A combination of equal parts of dried lemon balm, valerian root, and chamomile flowers should be prepared. Steep 1 teaspoon of the blend in 1 cup of hot water for 10 minutes. Strain and drink as needed.


## 36. Cold Sore Treatment Blend:

Ingredients: Lemon balm, licorice root, and echinacea.

Benefits: Lemon balm reduces cold sore outbreaks, licorice root heals, and echinacea boosts the immune system.

Recipe: Combine equal parts of dried lemon balm, licorice root, and echinacea. One teaspoon of the blend should be steeped in one cup of hot water for ten minutes. The solution should then be strained and consumed as required.


## 37. Inflammation Reduction Tea:

Ingredients: Turmeric, ginger, and boswellia.

Benefits: Turmeric and ginger reduce inflammation, and boswellia supports joint health.

Recipe: A combination of equal parts of dried turmeric root, ginger root, and boswellia should be prepared. One teaspoon of the aforementioned blend should be simmered in one cup of water for a period of ten minutes. The mixture should be strained and consumed twice daily.

**38. Hormone Balancing Blend:**

Ingredients: Vitex, black cohosh, and dong quai.

Benefits: Vitex regulates hormones, black cohosh alleviates menopause symptoms, and dong quai balances female hormones.

Recipe: Combine equal parts of dried vitex, black cohosh, and dong quai. Steep 1 teaspoon of the blend in 1 cup of hot water for 10 minutes. Strain and drink twice daily.

**39. Constipation Relief Tea:**

Ingredients: Senna, licorice root, and fennel.

Benefits: Senna promotes bowel movements, licorice root soothes the digestive tract, and fennel relieves gas.

Recipe: A combination of equal parts of dried senna leaves, liquorice root, and fennel seeds should be prepared. Steep 1 teaspoon of the blend in 1 cup of hot water for 10 minutes. Strain and drink as needed.

**40. Blood Sugar Balancing Blend:**

Ingredients: Cinnamon, fenugreek, and gymnema.

Benefits: Cinnamon helps regulate blood sugar, fenugreek improves insulin sensitivity, and gymnema reduces sugar cravings.

Recipe: Combine equal parts of dried cinnamon bark, fenugreek seeds, and gymnema. One teaspoon of the blend should be steeped in one cup of hot water for ten minutes. The solution should be strained and consumed twice daily.

### 41. Heart Support Tea:

Ingredients: Hawthorn, motherwort, and rose hips.

Benefits: Hawthorn strengthens the heart, motherwort calms the heart, and rose hips provide antioxidants.

Recipe: A combination of equal parts of dried hawthorn berries, motherwort, and rose hips should be prepared. One teaspoon of the blend should be steeped in one cup of hot water for ten minutes. The mixture should be strained and consumed on an as-needed basis.

### 42. Immune Strengthening Tea:

Ingredients: Astragalus, reishi, and ginger.

Benefits: Astragalus has been demonstrated to enhance immunity, reishi has been shown to promote overall health, and ginger has been found to possess anti-inflammatory properties.

Recipe: Combine equal parts of dried astragalus root, reishi mushroom, and ginger root. Simmer 1 tablespoon of the blend in 2 cups of water for 15 minutes. Strain and drink 1-2 cups daily.

### 43. Digestive Comfort Tea:

Ingredients: Chamomile, peppermint, and ginger.

Benefits: Chamomile soothes the digestive tract, peppermint relieves gas, and ginger reduces inflammation.

Recipe: A combination of equal parts of dried chamomile flowers, peppermint leaves, and ginger root should be prepared. Steep 1 teaspoon of the blend in 1 cup of hot water for 10 minutes. Strain and drink after meals.

## 44. Mood Uplifting Blend:

Ingredients: St. John's wort, lemon balm, and lavender.

Benefits: St. John's wort lifts mood, lemon balm calms, and lavender relaxes.

Recipe: Combine equal parts of dried St. John's wort, lemon balm, and lavender flowers. One teaspoon of the blend should be steeped in one cup of hot water for ten minutes. The solution should be strained and consumed on a daily basis.

## 45. Brain Health Tea:

Ingredients: Ginkgo biloba, gotu kola, and rosemary.

Benefits: Ginkgo biloba improves circulation to the brain, gotu kola enhances cognitive function, and rosemary boosts memory.

Recipe: The proportions of the ingredients should be equal, with the addition of dried ginkgo biloba leaves, gotu kola, and rosemary. One teaspoon of the blend should be steeped in one cup of hot water for ten minutes. The solution should be strained and consumed on a daily basis.

## 46. Relaxation Tea:

Ingredients: Valerian, chamomile, and hops.

Benefits: Valerian is known to promote relaxation, while chamomile is used to soothe and hops are employed to calm the mind.

Recipe: Combine equal parts of dried valerian root, chamomile flowers, and hops. Steep 1 teaspoon of the blend in 1 cup of hot water for 10 minutes. Strain and drink before bedtime.

## 47. Cold Prevention Blend:

Ingredients: Echinacea, elderberry, and rose hips.

Benefits: Echinacea boosts immunity, elderberry fights infections, and rose hips provide vitamin C.

Recipe: A combination of equal parts of dried echinacea root, elderberries, and rose hips should be prepared. Simmer 1 tablespoon of the blend in 2 cups of water for 15 minutes. Strain and drink 1-2 cups daily during cold season.


## 48. Stomach Soothing Tea:

Ingredients: Marshmallow root, slippery elm, and peppermint.

Benefits: Marshmallow root soothes the digestive tract, slippery elm coats the stomach lining, and peppermint relieves gas.

Recipe: Combine equal parts of dried marshmallow root, slippery elm, and peppermint leaves. One teaspoon of the blend should be steeped in one cup of hot water for ten minutes. The solution should then be strained and consumed as required.


## 49. Cholesterol Lowering Blend:

Ingredients: Artichoke leaf, fenugreek, and garlic.

Benefits: Artichoke leaf lowers cholesterol, fenugreek improves lipid profiles, and garlic supports heart health.

Recipe: A combination of equal parts of dried artichoke leaf, fenugreek seeds, and garlic should be prepared. One teaspoon of the blend should be steeped in one cup of hot water for ten minutes. The mixture should be strained and consumed on an as-needed basis.

### 50. Post-Workout Recovery Tea:

Ingredients: Turmeric, ginger, and nettle.

Benefits: The incorporation of turmeric and ginger into a dietary regimen can serve to reduce inflammation, while the consumption of nettle can facilitate the replenishment of nutrients essential for muscle recovery.

Recipe: Combine equal parts of dried turmeric root, ginger root, and nettle leaves. Simmer 1 teaspoon of the blend in 1 cup of water for 10 minutes. Strain and drink after workouts.

### 51. Respiratory Relief Blend:

Ingredients: Mullein, licorice root, and thyme.

Benefits: Mullein soothes the respiratory tract, licorice root heals, and thyme acts as an antimicrobial.

Recipe: A combination of equal parts of dried mullein leaves, licorice root, and thyme should be prepared. Steep 1 teaspoon of the blend in 1 cup of hot water for 10 minutes. Strain and drink twice daily.

### 52. Bone Density Support Tea:

Ingredients: Horsetail, nettle, and oat straw.

Benefits: Horsetail provides silica, nettle offers minerals, and oat straw supports bone health.

Recipe: Combine equal parts of dried horsetail, nettle, and oat straw. One teaspoon of the blend should be steeped in one cup of hot water for ten minutes. The solution should be strained and consumed on a daily basis.

## 53. Vision Support Blend:

Ingredients: Bilberry, eyebright, and goji berry.

Benefits: Bilberry supports eye health, eyebright soothes, and goji berry provides antioxidants.

Recipe: A suitable proportion of the ingredients is to be combined, namely equal parts of dried bilberry leaves, eyebright, and goji berries. One teaspoon of the blend should be steeped in one cup of hot water for ten minutes. The mixture should be strained and consumed on an as-needed basis.

## 54. Immune Enhancer Tea:

Ingredients: Astragalus, echinacea, and reishi.

Benefits: Astragalus has been demonstrated to enhance immunity, echinacea has been shown to fight infections, and reishi has been found to enhance overall health.

Recipe: Combine equal parts of dried astragalus root, echinacea root, and reishi mushroom. Simmer 1 tablespoon of the blend in 2 cups of water for 15 minutes. Strain and drink 1-2 cups daily.

## 55. Digestive Calm Tea:

Ingredients: Chamomile, peppermint, and fennel.

Benefits: Chamomile soothes the digestive tract, peppermint relieves gas, and fennel reduces bloating.

Recipe: A combination of equal parts of dried chamomile flowers, peppermint leaves, and fennel seeds should be prepared. Steep 1 teaspoon of the blend in 1 cup of hot water for 10 minutes. Strain and drink after meals.

## 56. Mood Booster Blend:

Ingredients: St. John's wort, lemon balm, and saffron.

Benefits: St. John's wort lifts mood, lemon balm calms, and saffron boosts serotonin levels.

Recipe: Combine equal parts of dried St. John's wort, lemon balm, and saffron. One teaspoon of the blend should be steeped in one cup of hot water for ten minutes. The solution should be strained and consumed on a daily basis.

## 57. Brain Function Tea:

Ingredients: Ginkgo biloba, gotu kola, and rosemary.

Benefits: Ginkgo biloba improves circulation to the brain, gotu kola enhances cognitive function, and rosemary boosts memory.

Recipe: The proportions of the ingredients should be equal, with the addition of dried ginkgo biloba leaves, gotu kola, and rosemary. One teaspoon of the blend should be steeped in one cup of hot water for ten minutes. The solution should be strained and consumed on a daily basis.

## 58. Relaxation and Sleep Blend:

Ingredients: Valerian, chamomile, and hops.

Benefits: Valerian is known to promote relaxation, while chamomile is used to soothe, and hops are employed to calm the mind.

Recipe: Combine equal parts of dried valerian root, chamomile flowers, and hops. Steep 1 teaspoon of the blend in 1 cup of hot water for 10 minutes. Strain and drink before bedtime.

## 59. Cold Defense Tea:

Ingredients: Echinacea, elderberry, and rose hips.

Benefits: Echinacea boosts immunity, elderberry fights infections, and rose hips provide vitamin C.

Recipe: A combination of equal parts of dried echinacea root, elderberries, and rose hips should be prepared. Simmer 1 tablespoon of the blend in 2 cups of water for 15 minutes. Strain and drink 1-2 cups daily during cold season.

## 60. Stomach Soothing Blend:

Ingredients: Marshmallow root, slippery elm, and peppermint.

Benefits: Marshmallow root soothes the digestive tract, slippery elm coats the stomach lining, and peppermint relieves gas.

Recipe: Combine equal parts of dried marshmallow root, slippery elm, and peppermint leaves. One teaspoon of the blend should be steeped in one cup of hot water for ten minutes. The solution should then be strained and consumed as required.

### Recipes of Synergistic Blends

Synergistic blends are meticulously crafted combinations of herbs that work in concert to amplify each other's effects. The following paragraphs will present a series of detailed examples:

### 61. Calming Sleep Tonic:

Ingredients: Valerian root, passionflower, lemon balm, and hops.

Benefits: Valerian root and passionflower are potent relaxants, lemon balm soothes the nervous system, and hops promotes restful sleep.

Recipe: A combination of equal parts of dried valerian root, passionflower, lemon balm, and hops should be prepared. One tablespoon of the blend should be steeped in one cup of hot water for 15 minutes. The mixture should then be strained and consumed approximately 30 minutes prior to bedtime.

### 62. Anti-Inflammatory Blend:

Ingredients: Turmeric, ginger, boswellia, and black pepper.

Benefits: The spices turmeric and boswellia have anti-inflammatory properties, ginger enhances circulation and has anti-inflammatory properties, and black pepper increases the bioavailability of turmeric.

Recipe: Combine 2 parts turmeric powder, 1 part ginger powder, 1 part boswellia powder, and a pinch of black pepper. Mix well. Take 1 teaspoon of the blend mixed with honey or in warm water once daily.

## 63. *Digestive Comfort Blend:*

Ingredients: Peppermint, ginger, chamomile, and fennel.

Benefits: Peppermint soothes the digestive tract, ginger reduces nausea, chamomile calms the stomach, and fennel relieves gas and bloating.

Recipe: A combination of equal parts of dried peppermint leaves, ginger root, chamomile flowers, and fennel seeds should be prepared. Steep 1 teaspoon of the blend in 1 cup of hot water for 10 minutes. Strain and drink after meals.

## 64. *Immune Support Blend:*

Ingredients: Echinacea, elderberry, astragalus, and rose hips.

Benefits: Echinacea boosts the immune system, elderberry fights infections, astragalus enhances vitality, and rose hips provide vitamin C.

Recipe: Combine equal parts of dried echinacea root, elderberries, astragalus root, and rose hips. One tablespoon of the blend should be simmered in two cups of water for approximately fifteen minutes. The resulting liquid should be strained and consumed in quantities of one to two cups per day.

## 65. *Respiratory Relief Blend:*

Ingredients: Mullein, thyme, elecampane, and licorice root.

Benefits: Mullein soothes the respiratory tract, thyme acts as an antimicrobial, elecampane supports lung health, and licorice root heals and soothes.

Recipe: A combination of equal parts of dried mullein leaves, thyme, elecampane root, and licorice root should be prepared. One teaspoon of the blend should be steeped in one cup of hot water for ten minutes. The solution should be strained and consumed twice daily.

## 66. Detoxifying Blend:

Ingredients: Dandelion root, burdock root, red clover, and nettle.

Benefits: Dandelion root and burdock root facilitate the detoxification of the liver, red clover acts as a blood purifier, and nettle provides essential nutrients.

Recipe: Combine equal parts of dried dandelion root, burdock root, red clover, and nettle leaves. Steep 1 teaspoon of the blend in 1 cup of hot water for 10 minutes. Strain and drink once daily.

## 67. Hormone Balance Blend:

Ingredients: Vitex, red clover, dong quai, and licorice root.

Benefits: Vitex regulates hormones, red clover supports menopause symptoms, dong quai balances female hormones, and licorice root acts as an adaptogen.

Recipe: A combination of equal parts of dried vitex berries, red clover, dong quai root, and licorice root should be prepared. Steep 1 teaspoon of the blend in 1 cup of hot water for 10 minutes. Strain and drink twice daily.

## 68. Energy Boosting Blend:

Ingredients: Ginseng, green tea, gotu kola, and peppermint.

Benefits: Ginseng boosts energy, green tea provides antioxidants and a gentle caffeine boost, gotu kola enhances cognitive function, and peppermint invigorates.

Recipe: Combine equal parts of dried ginseng root, green tea leaves, gotu kola, and peppermint leaves. One teaspoon of the blend should be steeped in one cup of hot water for a period of five minutes. The mixture should then be strained and consumed in the morning.


## 69. Skin Healing Blend:

Ingredients: Calendula, chamomile, lavender, and comfrey.

Benefits: Calendula promotes skin healing, chamomile soothes inflammation, lavender has antimicrobial properties, and comfrey supports tissue repair.

Recipe: A combination of equal parts of dried calendula flowers, chamomile flowers, lavender flowers, and comfrey root should be prepared. One teaspoon of the blend should be steeped in one cup of hot water for ten minutes. The resulting solution should be strained and applied as a wash or consumed as a drink once daily.


## 70. Heart Health Blend:

Ingredients: Hawthorn, motherwort, hibiscus, and ginger.

Benefits: Hawthorn has been demonstrated to strengthen the heart, while motherwort has been shown to calm the heart. Hibiscus has been found to lower blood pressure, and ginger has been proven to improve circulation.

Recipe: Combine equal parts of dried hawthorn berries, motherwort, hibiscus flowers, and ginger root. Steep 1 teaspoon of the blend in 1 cup of hot water for 10 minutes. Strain and drink once daily.

## 71. Anti-Anxiety Blend:

Ingredients: Lemon balm, valerian, passionflower, and lavender.

Benefits: Lemon balm calms the mind, valerian reduces anxiety, passionflower promotes relaxation, and lavender soothes.

Recipe: A combination of equal parts of dried lemon balm leaves, valerian root, passionflower, and lavender flowers should be prepared. Steep 1 teaspoon of the blend in 1 cup of hot water for 10 minutes. Strain and drink as needed.

## 72. Cold and Flu Blend:

Ingredients: Elderflower, yarrow, peppermint, and echinacea.

Benefits: Elderflower boosts the immune system, yarrow reduces fever, peppermint soothes respiratory symptoms, and echinacea fights infections.

Recipe: Combine equal parts of dried elderflower, yarrow, peppermint leaves, and echinacea root. One teaspoon of the blend should be steeped in one cup of hot water for ten minutes. The solution should be strained and consumed two to three times daily during the course of the illness.

## 73. Digestive Aid Blend:

Ingredients: Peppermint, fennel, ginger, and licorice root.

Benefits: Peppermint soothes the digestive tract, fennel relieves gas, ginger reduces nausea, and licorice root heals and soothes.

Recipe: A suitable proportion of the ingredients is to be combined, namely equal parts of dried peppermint leaves, fennel seeds, ginger root, and licorice root. One teaspoon of the blend should be steeped in one cup of hot water for ten minutes. The mixture should then be strained and consumed after meals.


## 74. Anti-Nausea Blend:

Ingredients: Ginger, peppermint, fennel, and chamomile.

Benefits: Ginger has been demonstrated to reduce nausea, peppermint to relieve flatulence, fennel to soothe the digestive tract, and chamomile to calm the stomach.

Recipe: Combine equal parts of dried ginger root, peppermint leaves, fennel seeds, and chamomile flowers. Steep 1 teaspoon of the blend in 1 cup of hot water for 10 minutes. Strain and drink as needed.


## 75. Joint Health Blend:

Ingredients: Turmeric, ginger, boswellia, and black pepper.

Benefits: Turmeric and boswellia reduce inflammation, ginger enhances circulation, and black pepper increases the bioavailability of turmeric.

Recipe: The ingredients should be combined in the following proportions: two parts turmeric powder, one part ginger powder, one part boswellia powder, and a pinch of black pepper. Mix well. Take 1 teaspoon of the blend mixed with honey or in warm water once daily.

## 76. Anti-Depression Blend:

Ingredients: St. John's wort, lemon balm, saffron, and rosemary.

Benefits: St. John's wort lifts mood, lemon balm calms the mind, saffron boosts serotonin levels, and rosemary enhances cognitive function.

Recipe: Combine equal parts of dried St. John's wort, lemon balm leaves, saffron, and rosemary. One teaspoon of the blend should be steeped in one cup of hot water for ten minutes. The solution should be strained and consumed on a daily basis.

## 77. Cold Sore Blend:

Ingredients: Lemon balm, licorice root, echinacea, and peppermint.

Benefits: Lemon balm reduces cold sore outbreaks, licorice root heals, echinacea boosts the immune system, and peppermint soothes.

Recipe: A combination of equal parts of dried lemon balm, licorice root, echinacea root, and peppermint leaves should be prepared. One teaspoon of the blend should be steeped in one cup of hot water for ten minutes. The mixture should then be strained and consumed as needed.

## 78. Menstrual Relief Blend:

Ingredients: Red raspberry leaf, cramp bark, ginger, and chamomile.

Benefits: Red raspberry leaf has a uterotonic effect, cramp bark is analgesic and reduces menstrual cramps, ginger has anti-inflammatory properties, and chamomile has a soothing effect on the stomach.

Recipe: Combine equal parts of dried red raspberry leaf, cramp bark, ginger root, and chamomile flowers. Steep 1 teaspoon of the blend in 1 cup of hot water for 10 minutes. Strain and drink as needed.

## 79. Memory and Focus Blend:

Ingredients: Ginkgo biloba, rosemary, gotu kola, and peppermint.

Benefits: Ginkgo biloba improves circulation to the brain, rosemary enhances cognitive function, gotu kola supports mental clarity, and peppermint invigorates.

Recipe: A combination of equal parts of dried ginkgo biloba leaves, rosemary, gotu kola, and peppermint leaves should be prepared. Steep 1 teaspoon of the blend in 1 cup of hot water for 10 minutes. Strain and drink once daily.

## 80. Heartburn Relief Blend:

Ingredients: Marshmallow root, licorice root, slippery elm, and fennel.

Benefits: Marshmallow root soothes the digestive tract, licorice root heals, slippery elm coats the stomach lining, and fennel relieves gas.

Recipe: Combine equal parts of dried marshmallow root, licorice root, slippery elm, and fennel seeds. One teaspoon of the blend should be steeped in one cup of hot water for ten minutes. The solution should then be strained and consumed as required.

### 81. Sleep Aid Blend:

Ingredients: Valerian root, passionflower, lemon balm, and chamomile.

Benefits: Valerian root promotes relaxation, passionflower calms the mind, lemon balm soothes the nervous system, and chamomile aids sleep.

Recipe: A suitable proportion of the following ingredients should be combined: dried valerian root, passionflower, lemon balm leaves, and chamomile flowers. One tablespoon of the blend should be steeped in one cup of hot water for 15 minutes. The resulting infusion should be strained and consumed approximately 30 minutes prior to bedtime.

### 82. Weight Loss Support Blend:

Ingredients: Green tea, dandelion root, ginger, and cinnamon.

Benefits: Green tea has been demonstrated to enhance the metabolic rate, dandelion root has been shown to act as a diuretic, ginger has been found to reduce inflammation, and cinnamon has been proven to assist in regulating blood sugar.

Recipe: Combine equal parts of dried green tea leaves, dandelion root, ginger root, and cinnamon bark. Steep 1 teaspoon of the blend in 1 cup of hot water for 5 minutes. Strain and drink once daily.

### 83. Bone Health Blend:

Ingredients: Horsetail, nettle, oat straw, and red clover.

Benefits: Horsetail provides silica, nettle offers minerals, oat straw supports bone density, and red clover provides phytoestrogens.

Recipe: A combination of equal parts of dried horsetail, nettle leaves, oat straw, and red clover should be prepared. Steep 1 teaspoon of the blend in 1 cup of hot water for 10 minutes. Strain and drink once daily.


### 84. Kidney Support Blend:

Ingredients: Nettle, dandelion leaf, corn silk, and marshmallow root.

Benefits: Nettle supports kidney function, dandelion leaf acts as a diuretic, corn silk soothes the urinary tract, and marshmallow root heals and soothes.

Recipe: Combine equal parts of dried nettle leaves, dandelion leaf, corn silk, and marshmallow root. One teaspoon of the blend should be steeped in one cup of hot water for ten minutes. The solution should be strained and consumed twice daily.


### 85. Thyroid Support Blend:

Ingredients: Ashwagandha, bladderwrack, licorice root, and nettle.

Benefits: Ashwagandha supports thyroid function, bladderwrack provides iodine, licorice root balances hormones, and nettle provides nutrients.

Recipe: A combination of equal parts of dried ashwagandha root, bladderwrack, licorice root, and nettle leaves should be prepared. One teaspoon of the blend should be steeped in one cup of hot water for ten minutes. The resulting solution should be strained and consumed on a daily basis..

## 86. Diabetes Support Blend:

Ingredients: Cinnamon, fenugreek, gymnema, and bilberry.

Benefits: Cinnamon has been demonstrated to regulate blood sugar, fenugreek has been shown to improve insulin sensitivity, gymnema has been found to reduce sugar cravings, and bilberry has been proven to support eye health.

Recipe: Combine equal parts of dried cinnamon bark, fenugreek seeds, gymnema, and bilberry leaves. Steep 1 teaspoon of the blend in 1 cup of hot water for 10 minutes. Strain and drink twice daily.

## 87. Cholesterol Lowering Blend:

Ingredients: Artichoke leaf, fenugreek, garlic, and hibiscus.

Benefits: Artichoke leaf lowers cholesterol, fenugreek improves lipid profiles, garlic supports heart health, and hibiscus provides antioxidants.

Recipe: A combination of equal parts of dried artichoke leaf, fenugreek seeds, garlic, and hibiscus flowers should be prepared. Steep 1 teaspoon of the blend in 1 cup of hot water for 10 minutes. Strain and drink once daily.

## 88. Bone Density Support Blend:

Ingredients: Horsetail, nettle, oat straw, and red clover.

Benefits: Horsetail provides silica, nettle offers minerals, oat straw supports bone health, and red clover provides phytoestrogens.

Recipe: Combine equal parts of dried horsetail, nettle leaves, oat straw, and red clover. One teaspoon of the blend should be steeped in one cup of hot water for ten minutes. The solution should be strained and consumed on a daily basis.

## 89. Digestive Health Blend:

Ingredients: Dandelion root, burdock root, ginger, and peppermint.

Benefits: Dandelion root supports digestion, burdock root detoxifies, ginger reduces inflammation, and peppermint relieves gas.

Recipe: A combination of equal parts of dried dandelion root, burdock root, ginger root, and peppermint leaves should be prepared. One teaspoon of the blend should be simmered in one cup of water for ten minutes. The resulting liquid should be strained and consumed twice daily.

## 90. Memory Support Blend:

Ingredients: Ginkgo biloba, gotu kola, rosemary, and peppermint.

Benefits: Ginkgo biloba has been demonstrated to improve cerebral circulation, while gotu kola has been shown to enhance cognitive function. Rosemary has been found to boost memory, and peppermint has been shown to invigorate.

Recipe: Combine equal parts of dried ginkgo biloba leaves, gotu kola, rosemary, and peppermint leaves. Steep 1 teaspoon of the blend in 1 cup of hot water for 10 minutes. Strain and drink once daily.

## 91. Bone Strength Blend:

Ingredients: Horsetail, nettle, oat straw, and red clover.

Benefits: Horsetail provides silica, nettle offers minerals, oat straw supports bone density, and red clover provides phytoestrogens.

Recipe: The ingredients should be combined in equal parts, namely horsetail, nettle leaves, oat straw, and red clover. Steep 1 teaspoon of the blend in 1 cup of hot water for 10 minutes. Strain and drink once daily.


## 92. Respiratory Health Blend:

Ingredients: Mullein, thyme, elecampane, and licorice root.

Benefits: Mullein soothes the respiratory tract, thyme acts as an antimicrobial, elecampane supports lung health, and licorice root heals and soothes.

Recipe: Combine equal parts of dried mullein leaves, thyme, elecampane root, and licorice root. One teaspoon of the blend should be steeped in one cup of hot water for ten minutes. The solution should be strained and consumed twice daily.


## 93. Skin Health Blend:

Ingredients: Calendula, chamomile, lavender, and comfrey.

Benefits: Calendula promotes skin healing, chamomile soothes inflammation, lavender has antimicrobial properties, and comfrey supports tissue repair.

Recipe: A combination of equal parts of dried calendula flowers, chamomile flowers, lavender flowers, and comfrey root should be prepared. One teaspoon of the blend should be steeped in one cup of hot water for ten minutes. The resulting solution should be strained and applied as a wash or consumed as a drink once daily.

## 94. Immune Boosting Blend:

Ingredients: Echinacea, elderberry, astragalus, and ginger.

Benefits: Echinacea has been demonstrated to enhance the immune system, elderberry has been shown to fight infections, astragalus has been found to enhance vitality, and ginger has been proven to possess anti-inflammatory and warming properties.

Recipe: Combine equal parts of dried echinacea root, elderberries, astragalus root, and ginger root. Simmer 1 tablespoon of the blend in 2 cups of water for 15 minutes. Strain and drink 1-2 cups daily during cold and flu season.

## 95. Stress Relief Blend:

Ingredients: Ashwagandha, holy basil, and lemon balm.

Benefits: Ashwagandha helps reduce stress and anxiety, holy basil acts as an adaptogen to balance the body, and lemon balm promotes relaxation.

Recipe: A combination of equal parts of dried ashwagandha root, holy basil leaves, and lemon balm leaves should be prepared. Steep 1 teaspoon of the blend in 1 cup of hot water for 15 minutes. Strain and drink 1-2 times daily.

## 96. Digestive Aid Tea:

Ingredients: Peppermint, fennel, and chamomile.

Benefits: Peppermint soothes the digestive tract, fennel relieves gas and bloating, and chamomile calms and supports digestion.

Recipe: Combine equal parts of dried peppermint leaves, fennel seeds, and chamomile flowers. One teaspoon of the blend should be steeped in one cup of hot water for ten minutes. The mixture should then be strained and consumed following a meal.

## 97. Energy Boosting Tea:

Ingredients: Ginseng, green tea, and licorice root.

Benefits: Ginseng boosts energy levels, green tea provides a gentle caffeine boost and antioxidants, and licorice root supports adrenal health.

Recipe: A suitable proportion of the ingredients is to be combined in equal parts, namely dried ginseng root, green tea leaves, and liquorice root. One teaspoon of the aforementioned blend should be steeped in one cup of boiling water for a period of five minutes. The mixture should then be strained and consumed in the morning.

## 98. Anti-Inflammatory Tea:

Ingredients: Turmeric, ginger, and cinnamon.

Benefits: The incorporation of turmeric and ginger into a dietary regimen has been demonstrated to possess anti-inflammatory properties, while the inclusion of cinnamon has been shown to confer antioxidant benefits.

Recipe: Combine 2 parts turmeric root, 1 part ginger root, and 1 part cinnamon bark. Simmer 1 teaspoon of the blend in 1 cup of water for 10 minutes. Strain and drink twice daily.

## 99. Skin Healing Blend:

Ingredients: Calendula, chamomile, lavender, and comfrey.

Benefits: Calendula promotes skin healing, chamomile soothes inflammation, lavender has antimicrobial properties, and comfrey supports tissue repair.

Recipe: A combination of equal parts of dried calendula flowers, chamomile flowers, lavender flowers, and comfrey root should be prepared. Steep 1 teaspoon of the blend in 1 cup of hot water for 10 minutes. Strain and apply as a wash or drink once daily.


## 100. Heart Health Blend:

Ingredients: Hawthorn, motherwort, hibiscus, and ginger.

Benefits: Hawthorn strengthens the heart, motherwort calms the heart, hibiscus lowers blood pressure, and ginger improves circulation.

Recipe: Combine equal parts of dried hawthorn berries, motherwort, hibiscus flowers, and ginger root. One teaspoon of the blend should be steeped in one cup of hot water for ten minutes. The solution should be strained and consumed on a daily basis.


## 101. Anti-Anxiety Blend:

Ingredients: Lemon balm, valerian, passionflower, and lavender.

Benefits: Lemon balm calms the mind, valerian reduces anxiety, passionflower promotes relaxation, and lavender soothes.

Recipe: A suitable proportion of the ingredients is to be combined, namely equal parts of dried lemon balm leaves, valerian root, passionflower, and lavender flowers. One teaspoon of the blend should be steeped in one cup of hot water for ten minutes. The solution should then be strained and consumed as required.

## 102. Cold and Flu Blend:

Ingredients: Elderflower, yarrow, peppermint, and echinacea.

Benefits: Elderflower has been demonstrated to enhance the immune system, yarrow has been shown to reduce fever, peppermint has been found to alleviate respiratory symptoms, and echinacea has been proven to combat infections.

Recipe: Combine equal parts of dried elderflower, yarrow, peppermint leaves, and echinacea root. Steep 1 teaspoon of the blend in 1 cup of hot water for 10 minutes. Strain and drink 2-3 times daily during illness.

## 103. Digestive Aid Blend:

Ingredients: Peppermint, fennel, ginger, and licorice root.

Benefits: Peppermint soothes the digestive tract, fennel relieves gas, ginger reduces nausea, and licorice root heals and soothes.

Recipe: A combination of equal parts of dried peppermint leaves, fennel seeds, ginger root, and licorice root should be prepared. Steep 1 teaspoon of the blend in 1 cup of hot water for 10 minutes. Strain and drink after meals.

### 104. Anti-Nausea Blend:

Ingredients: Ginger, peppermint, fennel, and chamomile.

Benefits: Ginger reduces nausea, peppermint relieves gas, fennel soothes the digestive tract, and chamomile calms the stomach.

Recipe: Combine equal parts of dried ginger root, peppermint leaves, fennel seeds, and chamomile flowers. One teaspoon of the blend should be steeped in one cup of hot water for ten minutes. The solution should then be strained and consumed as required.

### 105. Joint Health Blend:

Ingredients: Turmeric, ginger, boswellia, and black pepper.

Benefits: Turmeric and boswellia reduce inflammation, ginger enhances circulation, and black pepper increases the bioavailability of turmeric.

Recipe: The ingredients should be combined in the following proportions: two parts turmeric powder, one part ginger powder, one part boswellia powder, and a pinch of black pepper. The mixture should be thoroughly combined. One teaspoon of the aforementioned blend, mixed with honey or in warm water, should be consumed on a daily basis.

### 106. Anti-Depression Blend:

Ingredients: St. John's wort, lemon balm, saffron, and rosemary.

Benefits: St. John's wort has been demonstrated to have an antidepressant effect, lemon balm has been shown to have a calming effect on the mind, saffron has been found to increase serotonin levels, and rosemary has been shown to enhance cognitive function.

Recipe: Combine equal parts of dried St. John's wort, lemon balm leaves, saffron, and rosemary. Steep 1 teaspoon of the blend in 1 cup of hot water for 10 minutes. Strain and drink once daily.

### 107. Cold Sore Blend:

Ingredients: Lemon balm, licorice root, echinacea, and peppermint.

Benefits: Lemon balm reduces cold sore outbreaks, licorice root heals, echinacea boosts the immune system, and peppermint soothes.

Recipe: A combination of equal parts of dried lemon balm, licorice root, echinacea root, and peppermint leaves should be prepared. Steep 1 teaspoon of the blend in 1 cup of hot water for 10 minutes. Strain and drink as needed.

### 108. Menstrual Relief Blend:

Ingredients: Red raspberry leaf, cramp bark, ginger, and chamomile.

Benefits: Red raspberry leaf tones the uterus, cramp bark relieves menstrual cramps, ginger reduces inflammation, and chamomile calms the stomach.

Recipe: Combine equal parts of dried red raspberry leaf, cramp bark, ginger root, and chamomile flowers. One teaspoon of the blend should be steeped in one cup of hot water for ten minutes. The solution should then be strained and consumed as required.

## 109. Memory and Focus Blend:

Ingredients: Ginkgo biloba, rosemary, gotu kola, and peppermint.

Benefits: Ginkgo biloba improves circulation to the brain, rosemary enhances cognitive function, gotu kola supports mental clarity, and peppermint invigorates.

Recipe: A suitable proportion of the ingredients is to be combined, namely equal parts of dried ginkgo biloba leaves, rosemary, gotu kola, and peppermint leaves. One teaspoon of the blend should be steeped in one cup of hot water for ten minutes. The solution should be strained and consumed on a daily basis.

## 110. Heartburn Relief Blend:

Ingredients: Marshmallow root, licorice root, slippery elm, and fennel.

Benefits: The marshmallow root has been demonstrated to have soothing effects on the digestive tract, while the licorice root has been shown to possess healing properties. The slippery elm, in turn, has been found to coat the stomach lining, and fennel has been observed to relieve gas.

Recipe: Combine equal parts of dried marshmallow root, licorice root, slippery elm, and fennel seeds. Steep 1 teaspoon of the blend in 1 cup of hot water for 10 minutes. Strain and drink as needed.

## 111. Sleep Aid Blend:

Ingredients: Valerian root, passionflower, lemon balm, and chamomile.

Benefits: Valerian root promotes relaxation, passionflower calms the mind, lemon balm soothes the nervous system, and chamomile aids sleep.

Recipe: A combination of equal parts of dried valerian root, passionflower, lemon balm leaves, and chamomile flowers should be prepared. Steep 1 tablespoon of the blend in 1 cup of hot water for 15 minutes. Strain and drink 30 minutes before bedtime.

### 112. Weight Loss Support Blend:

Ingredients: Green tea, dandelion root, ginger, and cinnamon.

Benefits: Green tea boosts metabolism, dandelion root acts as a diuretic, ginger reduces inflammation, and cinnamon helps regulate blood sugar.

Recipe: Combine equal parts of dried green tea leaves, dandelion root, ginger root, and cinnamon bark. One teaspoon of the blend should be steeped in one cup of hot water for a period of five minutes. The solution should be strained and consumed on a daily basis.

### 113. Bone Health Blend:

Ingredients: Horsetail, nettle, oat straw, and red clover.

Benefits: Horsetail provides silica, nettle offers minerals, oat straw supports bone density, and red clover provides phytoestrogens.

Recipe: The ingredients should be combined in equal parts, namely dried horsetail, nettle leaves, oat straw, and red clover. One teaspoon of the blend should be steeped in one cup of hot water for ten minutes. The mixture should then be strained and consumed on an as-needed basis.

### 114. Kidney Support Blend:

Ingredients: Nettle, dandelion leaf, corn silk, and marshmallow root.

Benefits: Nettle has been demonstrated to support kidney function, dandelion leaf acts as a diuretic, corn silk soothes the urinary tract, and marshmallow root heals and soothes.

Recipe: Combine equal parts of dried nettle leaves, dandelion leaf, corn silk, and marshmallow root. Steep 1 teaspoon of the blend in 1 cup of hot water for 10 minutes. Strain and drink twice daily.

### 115. Thyroid Support Blend:

Ingredients: Ashwagandha, bladderwrack, licorice root, and nettle.

Benefits: Ashwagandha supports thyroid function, bladderwrack provides iodine, licorice root balances hormones, and nettle provides nutrients.

Recipe: The desired result can be achieved by combining equal parts of the following ingredients: dried ashwagandha root, bladderwrack, licorice root, and nettle leaves. Steep 1 teaspoon of the blend in 1 cup of hot water for 10 minutes. Strain and drink once daily.

### 116. Diabetes Support Blend:

Ingredients: Cinnamon, fenugreek, gymnema, and bilberry.

Benefits: Cinnamon helps regulate blood sugar, fenugreek improves insulin sensitivity, gymnema reduces sugar cravings, and bilberry supports eye health.

Recipe: Combine equal parts of dried cinnamon bark, fenugreek seeds, gymnema, and bilberry leaves. One teaspoon of the blend should be steeped in one cup of hot water for ten minutes. The solution should be strained and consumed twice daily.

## 117. Cholesterol Lowering Blend:

Ingredients: Artichoke leaf, fenugreek, garlic, and hibiscus.

Benefits: Artichoke leaf lowers cholesterol, fenugreek improves lipid profiles, garlic supports heart health, and hibiscus provides antioxidants.

Recipe: A combination of equal parts of dried artichoke leaf, fenugreek seeds, garlic, and hibiscus flowers should be prepared. One teaspoon of the blend should be steeped in one cup of hot water for ten minutes. The mixture should be strained and consumed on an as-needed basis.

## 118. Bone Density Support Blend:

Ingredients: Horsetail, nettle, oat straw, and red clover.

Benefits: Horsetail provides silica, nettle offers minerals, oat straw supports bone health, and red clover provides phytoestrogens.

Recipe: Combine equal parts of dried horsetail, nettle leaves, oat straw, and red clover. Steep 1 teaspoon of the blend in 1 cup of hot water for 10 minutes. Strain and drink once daily.

## 119. Liver Detox Blend:

Ingredients: Milk thistle, dandelion root, turmeric, and burdock root.

Benefits: Milk thistle detoxifies and protects the liver, dandelion root supports liver function, turmeric reduces inflammation, and burdock root aids in overall cleansing.

Recipe: A combination of equal parts of dried milk thistle seeds, dandelion root, turmeric root, and burdock root should be prepared. Simmer 1 teaspoon of the blend in 1 cup of water for 10 minutes. Strain and drink once daily.

## 120. Cold Prevention Blend:

Ingredients: Echinacea, elderberry, rose hips, and ginger.

Benefits: Echinacea boosts immunity, elderberry fights infections, rose hips provide vitamin C, and ginger adds anti-inflammatory properties.

Recipe: Combine equal parts of dried echinacea root, elderberries, rose hips, and ginger root. One tablespoon of the blend should be simmered in two cups of water for fifteen minutes. The resulting liquid should be strained and consumed in quantities of one to two cups per day during the period of cold weather.

## Detailed Recipes for Specific Health Issues

The provision of detailed, step-by-step recipes ensures that users can confidently prepare and utilise herbal remedies for specific health issues.

## 121. Headache Relief Tea:

Ingredients: Feverfew, peppermint, and willow bark.

Benefits: Feverfew reduces the frequency and severity of migraines, peppermint alleviates headache pain, and willow bark has pain-relieving properties similar to aspirin.

Recipe: The desired ratio is two parts dried feverfew leaves, one part dried peppermint leaves, and one part willow bark. One teaspoon of the aforementioned blend should be steeped in one cup of boiling water for a period of ten minutes. The solution should be strained and consumed as needed for headache relief.

## 122. Respiratory Support Syrup:

Ingredients: Elderberry, thyme, and honey.

Benefits: Elderberry has been demonstrated to enhance the immune system and to combat respiratory infections. Thyme has been shown to possess antimicrobial properties and to support lung health. Honey has been found to have a soothing effect on the throat.

Recipe: Simmer 1 cup of dried elderberries and 1/2 cup of dried thyme in 4 cups of water until reduced by half. Strain the liquid and add 1 cup of honey. Stir well and store in a glass jar. Take 1 tablespoon daily or as needed for respiratory support.

## 123. Sore Throat Gargle:

Ingredients: Sage, salt, and apple cider vinegar.

Benefits: Sage has antimicrobial properties, salt helps to reduce swelling, and apple cider vinegar balances pH levels.

Recipe: In a one-cup volume of boiling water, add one tablespoon of dried sage. Steep for 10 minutes, strain, then add 1 teaspoon of salt and 1 tablespoon of apple cider vinegar. Gargle as needed.

## 124. Digestive Aid Capsules:

Ingredients: Ginger, peppermint, and slippery elm.

Benefits: Ginger reduces nausea, peppermint soothes the digestive tract, and slippery elm coats and protects the stomach lining.

Recipe: Mix equal parts of powdered ginger, peppermint, and slippery elm. Fill size 00 capsules with the mixture. It is recommended that one or two capsules be taken after meals, as needed.

## 125. Anti-Anxiety Tincture:

Ingredients: Valerian root, skullcap, and lavender.

Benefits: Valerian root and skullcap calm the nervous system, and lavender promotes relaxation.

Recipe: A suitable ratio for combining equal parts of dried valerian root, skullcap, and lavender is as follows: Subsequently, the mixture should be covered with a suitable alcohol, such as vodka or brandy, and allowed to rest for a period of four to six weeks, with occasional shaking. The solution should then be strained and a teaspoonful taken as required.

## 126. Allergy Relief Capsules:

Ingredients: Nettle, quercetin, and vitamin C powder.

Benefits: Nettle has been demonstrated to reduce the histamine response, while quercetin has been shown to stabilize mast cells. Vitamin C has been found to support the immune system.

Recipe: Mix equal parts of powdered nettle, quercetin, and vitamin C. Fill size 00 capsules with the mixture. Take 1-2 capsules daily during allergy season.

### 127. Insomnia Relief Tea:

Ingredients: Chamomile, passionflower, and lemon balm.

Benefits: Chamomile soothes and relaxes, passionflower calms the mind, and lemon balm reduces anxiety.

Recipe: A combination of equal parts of dried chamomile flowers, passionflower, and lemon balm should be prepared. Steep 1 teaspoon of the blend in 1 cup of hot water for 10 minutes. Strain and drink 30 minutes before bedtime.


### 128. Cold Sore Ointment:

Ingredients: Lemon balm, St. John's wort, and beeswax.

Benefits: Lemon balm reduces the severity of outbreaks, St. John's wort has antiviral properties, and beeswax forms a protective barrier.

Recipe: Infuse 1 cup of olive oil with 1/2 cup of dried lemon balm and 1/2 cup of dried St. John's wort for 2 weeks. The mixture should be strained and heated gently with 1/4 cup of beeswax until the wax has melted. The prepared mixture should be poured into suitable containers and applied to the affected area as required.


### 129. Arthritis Relief Salve:

Ingredients: Cayenne, ginger, and coconut oil.

Benefits: Cayenne and ginger reduce inflammation and pain, and coconut oil soothes the skin.

Recipe: One cup of coconut oil should be infused with 1/4 cup of dried cayenne pepper and 1/4 cup of dried ginger for a period of two weeks. The mixture should then be strained and stored in a jar. As needed, apply to painful joints.

### 130. Anti-Dandruff Shampoo:

Ingredients: Rosemary, tea tree oil, and apple cider vinegar.

Benefits: Rosemary has been demonstrated to stimulate hair growth, tea tree oil has antifungal properties, and apple cider vinegar has been shown to balance scalp pH.

Recipe: Brew 1 cup of strong rosemary tea. Add 10 drops of tea tree oil and 1/4 cup of apple cider vinegar. Use as a shampoo, massaging into the scalp and rinsing thoroughly.

### 131. Stomach Soothing Tea:

Ingredients: Marshmallow root, chamomile, and peppermint.

Benefits: Marshmallow root soothes the digestive tract, chamomile calms the stomach, and peppermint relieves gas.

Recipe: The proportions of the ingredients should be equal, with the addition of dried marshmallow root, chamomile flowers, and peppermint leaves. Steep 1 teaspoon of the blend in 1 cup of hot water for 10 minutes. Strain and drink as needed.

### 132. Cough Syrup:

Ingredients: Thyme, honey, and lemon.

Benefits: Thyme has antimicrobial properties, honey soothes the throat, and lemon provides vitamin C.

Recipe: Simmer 1 cup of dried thyme in 2 cups of water until reduced by half. One cup of honey and the juice of one lemon should be strained and added to the mixture. It is recommended that one tablespoon be taken as needed.

## 133. Hemorrhoid Relief Ointment:

Ingredients: Witch hazel, calendula, and beeswax.

Benefits: Witch hazel reduces swelling, calendula promotes healing, and beeswax forms a protective barrier.

Recipe: One cup of olive oil should be infused with half a cup of dried calendula for a period of two weeks. The mixture should then be strained and heated gently with 1/4 cup of beeswax until the wax has melted. Subsequently, 1/4 cup of witch hazel extract should be added. The mixture should then be poured into containers and applied as needed.

## 134. Immune Boosting Gummies:

Ingredients: Elderberry, gelatin, and honey.

Benefits: Elderberry has been demonstrated to enhance the immune system, gelatin has been shown to promote gut health, and honey has been found to possess antibacterial properties and to add sweetness to a beverage.

Recipe: Simmer 1 cup of dried elderberries in 2 cups of water until reduced by half. Strain and add 1/4 cup of honey. Dissolve 1/4 cup of gelatin in 1/4 cup of cold water, then mix into the elderberry liquid. Pour into molds and refrigerate until set. Take 1-2 gummies daily.

### 135. *Sinus Relief Inhaler:*

Ingredients: Eucalyptus, peppermint, and tea tree oil.

Benefits: Eucalyptus and peppermint clear the sinuses, and tea tree oil has antimicrobial properties.

Recipe: To create an inhaler containing essential oils, add 10 drops each of eucalyptus, peppermint, and tea tree oil. Inhale as needed to relieve sinus congestion.


### 136. *Sunburn Relief Spray:*

Ingredients: Aloe vera, lavender, and peppermint.

Benefits: Aloe vera soothes and heals sunburned skin, lavender reduces pain and inflammation, and peppermint cools.

Recipe: Mix 1/2 cup of aloe vera gel with 10 drops each of lavender and peppermint essential oils. The solution can be added to a spray bottle and applied to sunburned skin as needed.


### 137. *Urinary Tract Infection Tea:*

Ingredients: Uva ursi, cranberry, and marshmallow root.

Benefits: Uva ursi has antibacterial properties, cranberry prevents bacterial adhesion, and marshmallow root soothes the urinary tract.

Recipe: A combination of equal parts of dried uva ursi, cranberry, and marshmallow root should be prepared. One teaspoon of the blend should be steeped in one cup of hot water for ten minutes. The solution should be strained and consumed two to three times daily.

### 138. Eye Wash for Conjunctivitis:

Ingredients: Eyebright, chamomile, and saline solution.

Benefits: Eyebright has been demonstrated to be an effective treatment for eye irritation, while chamomile has been shown to possess anti-inflammatory properties. Saline is a cleansing agent that is commonly used in eye care.

Recipe: Brew 1 cup of strong chamomile tea with 1 tablespoon of dried eyebright. Strain and mix with 1 cup of sterile saline solution. Use as an eye wash as needed.


### 139. Gout Relief Capsules:

Ingredients: Devil's claw, turmeric, and ginger.

Benefits: Devil's claw reduces pain and inflammation, turmeric reduces uric acid levels, and ginger enhances circulation.

Recipe: A uniform mixture of powdered devil's claw, turmeric, and ginger should be prepared in equal proportions. Fill size 00 capsules with the mixture. Take 1-2 capsules as needed.


### 140. Nausea Relief Lozenges:

Ingredients: Ginger, peppermint, and honey.

Benefits: Ginger reduces nausea, peppermint relieves gas, and honey soothes the throat.

Recipe: Mix 1 tablespoon of powdered ginger and 1 tablespoon of powdered peppermint with 1/4 cup of honey. The mixture should be formed into small balls and allowed to dry. As needed, consume lozenges by sucking on them.

### 141. Varicose Vein Cream:

Ingredients: Horse chestnut, witch hazel, and coconut oil.

Benefits: Horse chestnut strengthens vein walls, witch hazel reduces swelling, and coconut oil moisturizes.

Recipe: One cup of coconut oil should be infused with half a cup of dried horse chestnut and half a cup of witch hazel for a period of two weeks. The mixture should then be strained and stored in a jar. As needed, apply to varicose veins.

### 142. Cold and Flu Tea:

Ingredients: Elderberry, echinacea, and peppermint.

Benefits: Elderberry has been demonstrated to enhance the immune system, echinacea has been shown to combat infections, and peppermint has been found to alleviate respiratory symptoms.

Recipe: Combine equal parts of dried elderberries, echinacea root, and peppermint leaves. Steep 1 teaspoon of the blend in 1 cup of hot water for 10 minutes. Strain and drink 2-3 times daily during illness.

### 143. Sleep Aid Capsules:

Ingredients: Valerian root, passionflower, and lemon balm.

Benefits: Valerian root promotes relaxation, passionflower calms the mind, and lemon balm reduces anxiety.

Recipe: A uniform mixture of powdered valerian root, passionflower, and lemon balm should be prepared in equal proportions. Fill size 00 capsules with the mixture. Take 1-2 capsules 30 minutes before bedtime.

### 144. Skin Rash Ointment:

Ingredients: Calendula, chamomile, and beeswax.

Benefits: Calendula promotes healing, chamomile soothes inflammation, and beeswax forms a protective barrier.

Recipe: Infuse 1 cup of olive oil with 1/2 cup of dried calendula and 1/2 cup of dried chamomile for 2 weeks. The mixture should be strained and heated gently with 1/4 cup of beeswax until the wax has melted. The solution should then be poured into suitable containers and applied to the affected area as required..


### 145. Diarrhea Relief Tea:

Ingredients: Blackberry leaf, chamomile, and peppermint.

Benefits: Blackberry leaf astringes and reduces diarrhea, chamomile soothes the digestive tract, and peppermint relieves gas.

Recipe: A suitable proportion of the ingredients is to be combined, namely equal parts of dried blackberry leaf, chamomile flowers, and peppermint leaves. One teaspoon of the blend should be steeped in one cup of hot water for ten minutes. The solution should then be strained and consumed as required.


### 146. Allergy Relief Tea:

Ingredients: Nettle, peppermint, and elderflower.

Benefits: Nettle has been demonstrated to reduce the histamine response, peppermint has been shown to clear the sinuses, and elderflower has been found to boost the immune system.

Recipe: Combine equal parts of dried nettle leaves, peppermint leaves, and elderflowers. Steep 1 teaspoon of the blend in 1 cup of hot water for 10 minutes. Strain and drink as needed.

### 147. Eczema Relief Cream:

Ingredients: Calendula, chamomile, and coconut oil.

Benefits: Calendula promotes healing, chamomile reduces inflammation, and coconut oil moisturizes.

Recipe: One cup of coconut oil should be infused with half a cup of dried calendula and half a cup of dried chamomile for a period of two weeks. Strain and store in a jar. Apply to eczema as needed.

### 148. Cold Sore Lip Balm:

Ingredients: Lemon balm, St. John's wort, and beeswax.

Benefits: Lemon balm reduces the severity of outbreaks, St. John's wort has antiviral properties, and beeswax forms a protective barrier.

Recipe: Infuse 1 cup of olive oil with 1/2 cup of dried lemon balm and 1/2 cup of dried St. John's wort for 2 weeks. The mixture should be strained and heated gently with 1/4 cup of beeswax until the wax has melted. The mixture should then be poured into lip balm tubes and applied as required.

### 149. Anti-Inflammatory Capsules:

Ingredients: Turmeric, ginger, and boswellia.

Benefits: Turmeric and boswellia reduce inflammation, and ginger enhances circulation.

Recipe: A uniform mixture of powdered turmeric, ginger, and boswellia should be prepared. The mixture should be filled into size 00 capsules. It is recommended that one to two capsules be taken daily.

### 150. Acne Treatment Gel:

Ingredients: Tea tree oil, aloe vera, and lavender.

Benefits: Tea tree oil is known to possess antibacterial properties, aloe vera is known to possess soothing and healing properties, and lavender is known to possess anti-inflammatory properties.

Recipe: Mix 1/4 cup of aloe vera gel with 10 drops of tea tree oil and 10 drops of lavender essential oil. Apply to acne-prone areas as needed.

### 151. Sore Muscle Rub:

Ingredients: Cayenne, ginger, and coconut oil.

Benefits: Cayenne and ginger reduce inflammation and pain, and coconut oil soothes the skin.

Recipe: One cup of coconut oil should be infused with 1/4 cup of dried cayenne pepper and 1/4 cup of dried ginger for a period of two weeks. Strain and store in a jar. Apply to sore muscles as needed.

### 152. Nausea Relief Tea:

Ingredients: Ginger, peppermint, and fennel.

Benefits: Ginger reduces nausea, peppermint relieves gas, and fennel soothes the digestive tract.

Recipe: Combine equal parts of dried ginger root, peppermint leaves, and fennel seeds. One teaspoon of the blend should be steeped in one cup of hot water for ten minutes. The solution should then be strained and consumed as required.

### 153. Cold and Flu Capsules:

Ingredients: Echinacea, elderberry, and garlic.

Benefits: Echinacea boosts the immune system, elderberry fights infections, and garlic has antimicrobial properties.

Recipe: A uniform mixture of powdered echinacea, elderberry, and garlic should be prepared. The mixture should be filled into size 00 capsules. Administer one to two capsules, two to three times per day, during the course of the illness.

### 154. Sleep Aid Capsules:

Ingredients: Valerian root, passionflower, and lemon balm.

Benefits: Valerian root has been demonstrated to promote relaxation, passionflower has been shown to calm the mind, and lemon balm has been found to reduce anxiety.

Recipe: Mix equal parts of powdered valerian root, passionflower, and lemon balm. Fill size 00 capsules with the mixture. Take 1-2 capsules 30 minutes before bedtime.

### 155. Heart Health Tea:

Ingredients: Hawthorn, motherwort, and hibiscus.

Benefits: Hawthorn strengthens the heart, motherwort calms the heart, and hibiscus lowers blood pressure.

Recipe: A combination of equal parts of dried hawthorn berries, motherwort, and hibiscus flowers should be prepared. Steep 1 teaspoon of the blend in 1 cup of hot water for 10 minutes. Strain and drink once daily.

### 156. Gout Relief Capsules:

Ingredients: Devil's claw, turmeric, and ginger.

Benefits: Devil's claw reduces pain and inflammation, turmeric reduces uric acid levels, and ginger enhances circulation.

Recipe: Mix equal parts of powdered devil's claw, turmeric, and ginger. The size 00 capsules should be filled with the aforementioned mixture. The dosage is to be determined by the patient, with a range of one to two capsules per instance of use.

### 157. Cold Sore Ointment:

Ingredients: Lemon balm, St. John's wort, and beeswax.

Benefits: Lemon balm reduces the severity of outbreaks, St. John's wort has antiviral properties, and beeswax forms a protective barrier.

Recipe: One cup of olive oil should be infused with half a cup of dried lemon balm and half a cup of dried St. John's wort for a period of two weeks. The mixture should then be strained and heated gently with 1/4 cup of beeswax until the wax has melted. The mixture should then be poured into suitable containers and applied to the affected area as required.

## 158. Arthritis Relief Salve:

Ingredients: Cayenne, ginger, and coconut oil.

Benefits: The application of cayenne and ginger has been demonstrated to reduce inflammation and pain, while the use of coconut oil has been shown to have a soothing effect on the skin.

Recipe: Infuse 1 cup of coconut oil with 1/4 cup of dried cayenne pepper and 1/4 cup of dried ginger for 2 weeks. Strain and store in a jar. Apply to painful joints as needed.

## 159. Anti-Dandruff Shampoo:

Ingredients: Rosemary, tea tree oil, and apple cider vinegar.

Benefits: Rosemary stimulates hair growth, tea tree oil has antifungal properties, and apple cider vinegar balances scalp pH.

Recipe: One cup of strong rosemary tea should be brewed. Subsequently, 10 drops of tea tree oil and 1/4 cup of apple cider vinegar should be added. Use as a shampoo, massaging into the scalp and rinsing thoroughly.

## 160. Sore Throat Gargle:

Ingredients: Sage, salt, and apple cider vinegar.

Benefits: Sage has antimicrobial properties, salt helps to reduce swelling, and apple cider vinegar balances pH levels.

Recipe: Combine 1 tablespoon of dried sage with 1 cup of hot water. The solution should be steeped for a period of 10 minutes, after which it should be strained. Thereafter, 1 teaspoon of salt and 1 tablespoon of apple cider vinegar should be added. It is recommended that the solution be gargled as needed.

## 161. Immune Boosting Gummies:

Ingredients: Elderberry, gelatin, and honey.

Benefits: Elderberry boosts the immune system, gelatin supports gut health, and honey adds sweetness and antibacterial properties.

Recipe: One cup of dried elderberries should be simmered in two cups of water until the volume is reduced by half. The mixture should then be strained and 1/4 cup of honey should be added. One-quarter cup of gelatin should be dissolved in one-quarter cup of cold water, and then the resulting solution should be incorporated into the elderberry liquid. The mixture should then be poured into molds and refrigerated until it has set. It is recommended that one to two gummies be consumed daily.

## 162. Sinus Relief Inhaler:

Ingredients: Eucalyptus, peppermint, and tea tree oil.

Benefits: Eucalyptus and peppermint are known to clear the sinuses, while tea tree oil has antimicrobial properties.

Recipe: Add 10 drops each of eucalyptus, peppermint, and tea tree oil to an essential oil inhaler. Inhale as needed to relieve sinus congestion.

## 163. Sunburn Relief Spray:

Ingredients: Aloe vera, lavender, and peppermint.

Benefits: Aloe vera soothes and heals sunburned skin, lavender reduces pain and inflammation, and peppermint cools.

Recipe: A solution of aloe vera gel and essential oils of lavender and peppermint should be prepared by mixing 1/2 cup of aloe vera gel with 10 drops of each essential oil. Add to a spray bottle and apply to sunburned skin as needed.

## 164. Urinary Tract Infection Tea:

Ingredients: Uva ursi, cranberry, and marshmallow root.

Benefits: Uva ursi has antibacterial properties, cranberry prevents bacterial adhesion, and marshmallow root soothes the urinary tract.

Recipe: Combine equal parts of dried uva ursi, cranberry, and marshmallow root. One teaspoon of the blend should be steeped in one cup of hot water for ten minutes. The solution should be strained and consumed two to three times daily.

## 165. Eye Wash for Conjunctivitis:

Ingredients: Eyebright, chamomile, and saline solution.

Benefits: Eyebright soothes eye irritation, chamomile reduces inflammation, and saline cleanses.

Recipe: One cup of strong chamomile tea should be brewed with one tablespoon of dried eyebright. The solution should then be strained and mixed with one cup of sterile saline solution. The solution may be used as an eye wash as needed.

## 166. Allergy Relief Capsules:

Ingredients: Nettle, quercetin, and vitamin C powder.

Benefits: Nettle has been demonstrated to reduce the histamine response, while quercetin has been shown to stabilize mast cells. Vitamin C has been found to support the immune system.

Recipe: Mix equal parts of powdered nettle, quercetin, and vitamin C. Fill size 00 capsules with the mixture. Take 1-2 capsules daily during allergy season.

## 167. Insomnia Relief Tea:

Ingredients: Chamomile, passionflower, and lemon balm.

Benefits: Chamomile soothes and relaxes, passionflower calms the mind, and lemon balm reduces anxiety.

Recipe: A combination of equal parts of dried chamomile flowers, passionflower, and lemon balm should be prepared. Steep 1 teaspoon of the blend in 1 cup of hot water for 10 minutes. Strain and drink 30 minutes before bedtime.

## 168. Skin Rash Ointment:

Ingredients: Calendula, chamomile, and beeswax.

Benefits: Calendula promotes healing, chamomile soothes inflammation, and beeswax forms a protective barrier.

Recipe: Infuse 1 cup of olive oil with 1/2 cup of dried calendula and 1/2 cup of dried chamomile for 2 weeks. The mixture should be strained and heated gently with 1/4 cup of beeswax until the wax has melted. The solution should then be poured into suitable containers and applied to the affected area as required.

### 169. Diarrhea Relief Tea:

Ingredients: Blackberry leaf, chamomile, and peppermint.

Benefits: Blackberry leaf astringes and reduces diarrhea, chamomile soothes the digestive tract, and peppermint relieves gas.

Recipe: A suitable proportion of the ingredients is to be combined, namely equal parts of dried blackberry leaf, chamomile flowers, and peppermint leaves. One teaspoon of the blend should be steeped in one cup of hot water for ten minutes. The solution should then be strained and consumed as required.

### 170. Allergy Relief Tea:

Ingredients: Nettle, peppermint, and elderflower.

Benefits: Nettle has been demonstrated to reduce the histamine response, peppermint has been shown to clear the sinuses, and elderflower has been found to boost the immune system.

Recipe: Combine equal parts of dried nettle leaves, peppermint leaves, and elderflowers. Steep 1 teaspoon of the blend in 1 cup of hot water for 10 minutes. Strain and drink as needed.

### 171. Eczema Relief Cream:

Ingredients: Calendula, chamomile, and coconut oil.

Benefits: Calendula promotes healing, chamomile reduces inflammation, and coconut oil moisturizes.

Recipe: One cup of coconut oil should be infused with half a cup of dried calendula and half a cup of dried chamomile for a period of two weeks. Strain and store in a jar. Apply to eczema as needed.


### 172. Cold Sore Lip Balm:

Ingredients: Lemon balm, St. John's wort, and beeswax.

Benefits: Lemon balm reduces the severity of outbreaks, St. John's wort has antiviral properties, and beeswax forms a protective barrier.

Recipe: Infuse 1 cup of olive oil with 1/2 cup of dried lemon balm and 1/2 cup of dried St. John's wort for 2 weeks. The mixture should be strained and heated gently with 1/4 cup of beeswax until the wax has melted. The mixture should then be poured into lip balm tubes and applied as required.


### 173. Anti-Inflammatory Capsules:

Ingredients: Turmeric, ginger, and boswellia.

Benefits: Turmeric and boswellia reduce inflammation, and ginger enhances circulation.

Recipe: A uniform mixture of powdered turmeric, ginger, and boswellia should be prepared. The mixture should be filled into size 00 capsules. It is recommended that one to two capsules be taken daily.

### 174. Acne Treatment Gel:

Ingredients: Tea tree oil, aloe vera, and lavender.

Benefits: Tea tree oil is known to possess antibacterial properties, aloe vera is known to possess soothing and healing properties, and lavender is known to possess anti-inflammatory properties.

Recipe: Mix 1/4 cup of aloe vera gel with 10 drops of tea tree oil and 10 drops of lavender essential oil. Apply to acne-prone areas as needed.

### 175. Sore Muscle Rub:

Ingredients: Cayenne, ginger, and coconut oil.

Benefits: Cayenne and ginger reduce inflammation and pain, and coconut oil soothes the skin.

Recipe: One cup of coconut oil should be infused with 1/4 cup of dried cayenne pepper and 1/4 cup of dried ginger for a period of two weeks. Strain and store in a jar. Apply to sore muscles as needed.

### 176. Nausea Relief Tea:

Ingredients: Ginger, peppermint, and fennel.

Benefits: Ginger reduces nausea, peppermint relieves gas, and fennel soothes the digestive tract.

Recipe: Combine equal parts of dried ginger root, peppermint leaves, and fennel seeds. One teaspoon of the blend should be steeped in one cup of hot water for ten minutes. The solution should then be strained and consumed as required.

## 177. Cold and Flu Capsules:

Ingredients: Echinacea, elderberry, and garlic.

Benefits: Echinacea boosts the immune system, elderberry fights infections, and garlic has antimicrobial properties.

Recipe: A uniform mixture of powdered echinacea, elderberry, and garlic should be prepared. The mixture should be filled into size 00 capsules. It is recommended that one to two capsules be taken twice daily during the course of the illness.


## 178. Sleep Aid Capsules:

Ingredients: Valerian root, passionflower, and lemon balm.

Benefits: Valerian root has been demonstrated to promote relaxation, passionflower has been shown to calm the mind, and lemon balm has been found to reduce anxiety.

Recipe: Mix equal parts of powdered valerian root, passionflower, and lemon balm. Fill size 00 capsules with the mixture. Take 1-2 capsules 30 minutes before bedtime.


## 179. Heart Health Tea:

Ingredients: Hawthorn, motherwort, and hibiscus.

Benefits: Hawthorn strengthens the heart, motherwort calms the heart, and hibiscus lowers blood pressure.

Recipe: A combination of equal parts of dried hawthorn berries, motherwort, and hibiscus flowers should be prepared. Steep 1 teaspoon of the blend in 1 cup of hot water for 10 minutes. Strain and drink once daily.

### 180. Digestive Health Tea:

Ingredients: Dandelion root, burdock root, ginger, and peppermint.

Benefits: Dandelion root supports digestion, burdock root detoxifies, ginger reduces inflammation, and peppermint relieves gas.

Recipe: Combine equal parts of dried dandelion root, burdock root, ginger root, and peppermint leaves. One teaspoon of the blend should be steeped in one cup of hot water for ten minutes. The solution should be strained and consumed twice daily.

I In Chapter 5, we will examine the integration of traditional herbal knowledge with modern scientific advancements. This chapter will examine the evolution of traditional practices for contemporary use, integrating modern science with ancient wisdom, addressing the root causes of ailments, and developing holistic treatment plans for various conditions. By integrating the traditional with the contemporary, one can develop effective, informed, and comprehensive approaches to health and wellness that are both timeless and relevant.

# Chapter 5: Modern Applications

As we examine the realm of modern applications, we investigate the potential for adapting and expanding traditional herbal knowledge to meet contemporary health needs. The integration of modern scientific insights with ancient practices not only enhances the effectiveness of herbal remedies but also ensures their relevance in today's healthcare landscape. This chapter is devoted to the examination of traditional knowledge in the context of contemporary use. It addresses the root causes of ailments and presents a systematic approach to the development of holistic treatment plans for various conditions.

## Evolving Traditional Knowledge for Contemporary Use

The efficacy and naturalistic approach to healing have enabled traditional herbal practices to withstand the test of time. Nevertheless, with the advent of scientific and technological advances, there is a substantial potential to enhance these practices. By integrating modern scientific knowledge with ancient wisdom, it is possible to optimize the use of herbal remedies and improve health outcomes.

### Integrating Modern Science with Ancient Practices

- The scientific validation of herbal remedies is a topic of considerable interest to researchers in the field of complementary and alternative medicine. Modern science has enabled us to comprehend the biochemical processes underlying numerous traditional herbal remedies. The results of research studies can be used to validate the efficacy of herbs and identify their active compounds, thereby ensuring their safe and effective use.

- o Example: Extensive research has been conducted on curcumin, the active compound in turmeric, with regard to its anti-inflammatory and antioxidant properties. The scientific literature provides substantial evidence to support the traditional use of curcumin for reducing inflammation and promoting overall health.

- Standardization and Quality Control: The advent of advanced analytical techniques has enabled the standardization of herbal products. It is of the utmost importance to ensure that the quality and potency of herbal remedies remain consistent in order to guarantee their reliable use.

  - o Example: Standardized extracts of ginkgo biloba are now available, providing a consistent dose of its active compounds for cognitive support.

- Innovative Delivery Methods: The advent of modern technology has facilitated the development of novel delivery methods for herbal remedies, which have been shown to enhance their absorption and effectiveness.

  - o Example: The use of liposomal delivery systems has been shown to enhance the bioavailability of certain herbal compounds, such as curcumin and quercetin, thereby increasing their efficacy.

## Addressing Root Causes of Ailments

A holistic approach to health is one that focuses on identifying and addressing the root causes of ailments, as opposed to merely treating symptoms. This approach frequently entails a combination of herbal remedies, lifestyle modifications, and other holistic practices.

- Personalized Health Assessments: It is of paramount importance to gain an understanding of an individual's unique health profile in order to identify the root causes of their health issues. This may entail an assessment of dietary habits, lifestyle, stress levels, and genetic predispositions.

    o Example: An individual with chronic digestive issues may benefit from a comprehensive assessment that includes dietary analysis, stress management techniques, and specific herbal remedies such as peppermint and chamomile.

- Functional Medicine Principles: Functional medicine is a systems-oriented approach that emphasizes the interconnectedness of the body's systems. The objective is to restore equilibrium and optimal functionality.

    o Example: For individuals with autoimmune conditions, a functional medicine approach may include the use of anti-inflammatory herbs such as turmeric and boswellia, in conjunction with dietary modifications and stress reduction techniques.

- Preventive Health Strategies: Prevention is a fundamental aspect of holistic health. The use of herbal remedies and lifestyle practices to maintain health and prevent disease represents a proactive approach to health maintenance.

  - Example: The incorporation of adaptogenic herbs, such as ashwagandha and holy basil, has been demonstrated to assist in the management of stress and the prevention of stress-related health issues.

## Holistic Treatment Plans for Various Conditions

The creation of comprehensive treatment plans necessitates the integration of herbal remedies with other holistic practices, thereby enabling the addressing of a wide range of health conditions.

- Digestive Health Plan:

  - Assessment: Identify dietary triggers, stress factors, and microbial imbalances.

  - Herbal Remedies: Use peppermint, ginger, and licorice root to soothe and heal the digestive tract.

  - Lifestyle Practices: Implement dietary changes, stress management techniques, and probiotics to support gut health.

- Cardiovascular Health Plan:

    o Assessment: Evaluate diet, exercise habits, and stress levels.

    o Herbal Remedies: Include hawthorn, garlic, and cayenne to support heart health and improve circulation.

    o Lifestyle Practices: Encourage a heart-healthy diet, regular exercise, and mindfulness practices to reduce stress.

- Immune Support Plan:

    o Assessment: Assess overall health, nutritional status, and exposure to stress.

    o Herbal Remedies: Use echinacea, elderberry, and astragalus to enhance immune function.

    o Lifestyle Practices: Promote a balanced diet, adequate sleep, and regular physical activity to strengthen the immune system.

- Stress and Anxiety Management Plan:

    o Assessment: Identify stressors, emotional health, and coping mechanisms.

    o Herbal Remedies: Incorporate adaptogens like ashwagandha, rhodiola, and calming herbs such as lemon balm and passionflower.

    o Lifestyle Practices: Practice mindfulness, meditation, and yoga to manage stress effectively.

In Chapter 6, we will examine the practical aspects of creating one's own natural remedies. This chapter will cover a range of topics related to the gathering and preparation of herbs, including best practices for foraging and harvesting, sustainable and ethical sourcing, and various preparation methods. Furthermore, the chapter will address various preparation methods, including stovetop techniques, no-cook methods, and the art of proportion and balance. Furthermore, we will examine infusion techniques and the significance of rituals and mindfulness in the preparation of herbal remedies. The objective of this chapter is to provide the reader with the necessary skills and knowledge to create potent and personalized herbal remedies at home.

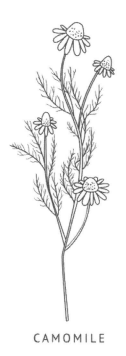

CAMOMILE

# Chapter 6: Creating Natural Remedies

The act of creating one's own natural remedies can be a rewarding and empowering experience. By acquiring an understanding of the most effective practices for foraging and harvesting herbs, and by mastering a range of preparation techniques, individuals can create effective and personalised herbal remedies. This chapter will guide the reader through the principles of sustainable and ethical sourcing, traditional stovetop methods, no-cook methods, the art of proportion and balance, infusion techniques, and the importance of rituals and mindfulness in remedy preparation.

## Best Practices for Foraging and Harvesting Herbs

The act of foraging and harvesting one's own herbs can facilitate a deeper connection with nature and ensure the use of the freshest and highest-quality ingredients in one's remedies. Nevertheless, it is of the utmost importance to adhere to principles of sustainability and ethical sourcing in order to safeguard the environment and guarantee the sustained availability of these invaluable resources.

### Sustainable and Ethical Sourcing

- **Identify Proper Locations**: Forage in areas that are free from pollution, pesticides, and other contaminants. Avoid roadsides and industrial areas.

- **Harvest Responsibly**: It is imperative that only the necessary amount of plant material be harvested, and that no more than a single plant or area be over-harvested. It is recommended that the rule of thirds be followed, whereby no more than one-third of any plant should be harvested at any one time, in order to allow it to continue growing and reproducing.

- **Respect Wildlife and Habitat**: Be mindful of the surrounding ecosystem and avoid disturbing wildlife habitats. Stick to established trails and avoid trampling vegetation.

- **Know Your Plants**: It is of the utmost importance to correctly identify each plant before harvesting, in order to prevent the collection of toxic or endangered species. Should uncertainty arise, it is advisable to consult field guides or to seek the advice of local experts.

- **Seasonal Awareness**: Harvest herbs during their peak seasons to ensure maximum potency and efficacy. Different plants have different optimal harvesting times, often related to their flowering or fruiting stages.

## Stovetop Methods

The preparation of herbal remedies by traditional stovetop methods has been employed for millennia and continues to be an effective means of extracting the medicinal properties of herbs.

- **Decoctions**: Used for tougher plant materials like roots, bark, and seeds.

    - Method: One to two tablespoons of the dried herb material should be placed in a pot with two cups of water. The mixture should then be brought to a boil, after which the heat should be reduced and the mixture simmered for a period of 20 to 30 minutes. The solution should then be strained and used as required.

- **Infusions**: Ideal for delicate plant parts like leaves and flowers.

  - Method: One tablespoon of the dried herb should be placed in a teapot or heatproof container. One cup of boiling water should be poured over the herbs, which should then be covered and steeped for 10-15 minutes. The resulting infusion should then be strained and utilized as needed.

## No-Cook Methods

No-cook methods provide convenient alternatives for preparing herbal remedies without the need for heat.

- **Tinctures**: Alcohol-based extracts that are easy to make and have a long shelf life.

  - Method: The jar should be filled to a depth of one-third of its capacity with dried herbs, or two-thirds of its capacity with fresh herbs. Subsequently, the jar should be covered with alcohol (vodka or brandy) in order to fill it. The jar should be sealed tightly and stored in a dark place for a period of 4-6 weeks, with occasional shaking. The solution should then be strained and stored in dark glass bottles..

- **Glycerites**: Glycerin-based extracts for those who prefer alcohol-free options.

    - Method: The jar should be filled to one-third of its capacity with dried herbs. The jar should then be covered with a mixture of three parts glycerin to one part water, in order to fill it. The jar should be sealed tightly and stored in a dark place for a period of 4-6 weeks, with occasional shaking. The solution should then be strained and stored in dark glass bottles.

- **Vinegars**: Herbal vinegars are both medicinal and culinary.

    - Method: The jar should be filled to one-third of its capacity with dried herbs. Subsequently, the jar should be covered with vinegar (apple cider vinegar is a commonly used option). The jar should be sealed tightly and stored in a dark place for a period of 4-6 weeks, with occasional shaking. Subsequently, the liquid should be strained and stored in dark glass bottles.

### The Art of Proportion and Balance

The creation of efficacious herbal remedies necessitates an appreciation of proportion and equilibrium. This ensures that the various herbs in a blend are compatible with one another and act in concert.

- **Primary Herbs**: These are the main herbs in a remedy, chosen for their specific therapeutic effects.

- **Supporting Herbs**: These herbs enhance the effects of the primary herbs and provide additional benefits.

- **Catalyst Herbs**: These herbs aid in the absorption and effectiveness of the primary and supporting herbs.

- **Proportions**: A typical ratio for herbal preparations might be 3 parts primary herbs, 2 parts supporting herbs, and 1 part catalyst herbs. It is recommended that the proportions be adjusted according to the specific needs and conditions of the individual.

## *Infusion Techniques*

Infusions are a key method for extracting the medicinal properties of herbs. There are several techniques to consider:

- **Cold Infusion**: Used for herbs that release their properties better in cold water, such as marshmallow root.
  - Method: One to two tablespoons of the desired dried herb should be placed in a jar. Subsequently, the mixture should be covered with cold water and allowed to steep overnight (between 8 and 12 hours). The resulting liquid should then be strained and used as needed.
- **Hot Infusion**: Commonly used for most herbs.
  - Method: One tablespoon of the dried herb should be placed in a teapot or heatproof container. One cup of boiling water should be poured over the herbs, which should then be covered and steeped for 10-15 minutes. The resulting infusion should then be strained and utilized as needed.
- **Sun Infusion**: Utilizes the energy of the sun to extract herbal properties.
  - Method: A jar should be filled with fresh herbs and then covered with water. The jar should then be sealed and placed in direct

sunlight for a period of 6-8 hours. The liquid should then be strained and used as required.

## Rituals and Mindfulness in Remedy Preparation

The incorporation of rituals and mindfulness into the preparation of herbal remedies has been demonstrated to enhance their effectiveness and facilitate a deeper connection with the healing process.

- *Mindful Gathering*: Approach foraging and harvesting with intention and gratitude. Take a moment to appreciate the plant and its environment.

- *Setting Intentions*: Before preparing a remedy, set a clear intention for its use. Focus on the desired outcome and visualize the healing process.

- *Creating a Sacred Space*: Prepare your remedies in a clean, quiet space free from distractions. Consider lighting a candle or playing soothing music.

- *Gratitude Practice*: Express gratitude for the plants and their healing properties. Acknowledge the interconnectedness of nature and your role in the healing process.

In Chapter 7, we will examine the potential of incorporating herbal remedies and holistic practices into one's daily routine to facilitate a healthier lifestyle. This chapter will address the integration of daily routines with natural cycles, seasonal health practices, daily self-care routines employing herbal remedies, nourishment beyond nutrition, incorporating movement and exercise into a holistic lifestyle, and building a deeper connection with nature. The integration of these practices allows for the creation of a balanced and harmonious approach to health and wellness, fostering a deeper connection with oneself and the natural world.

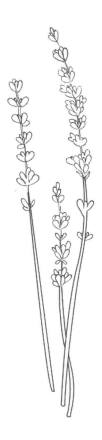

LAVENDER

# Chapter 7: Revitalize Your Routine: Embracing a Healthier Lifestyle

Embracing a healthier lifestyle necessitates more than merely sporadic wellness practices; it requires the integration of holistic habits into one's daily routine. This chapter will provide guidance on how to align one's daily activities with natural cycles, incorporate seasonal health practices, create daily self-care routines using herbal remedies, nourish the mind and spirit, include movement and exercise in a holistic manner, and build a deeper connection with nature.

## Aligning Daily Routines with Natural Cycles

An understanding and harmonization with the natural cycles of the day and year can enhance one's overall well-being. By aligning one's routines with these cycles, one can support the body's natural rhythms and promote balance and health.

### Seasonal Health Practices

Each season presents a unique set of challenges and opportunities for maintaining health. By modifying one's wellness practices to align with the seasonal changes, it is possible to maintain a balanced and vibrant state throughout the year.

- *Spring*:

Focus: Detoxification and renewal.

Practices: Incorporate herbs that facilitate detoxification, such as dandelion and nettle. It is recommended that individuals engage in gentle cleansing diets and increase physical activity in order to stimulate the body's natural detoxification processes.

- *Summer*:

Focus: Hydration and cooling.

Practices: It is recommended that cooling herbs such as peppermint and hibiscus be utilized. Consume light, hydrating foods such as fruits and vegetables. It is recommended that individuals engage in outdoor activities and ensure adequate hydration.

- *Autumn*:

Focus: Immunity and grounding.

Practices: It is recommended that the immune system be strengthened through the use of herbs such as elderberry and echinacea. Consume foods that are considered grounding and warming, such as root vegetables. It is recommended that individuals engage in mindfulness and reflection exercises in order to prepare for the introspective winter months.

- *Winter*:

Focus: Nourishment and rest.

Practices: It is recommended that nourishing herbs such as ashwagandha and astragalus be incorporated into one's diet. It is recommended that individuals consume warming, hearty foods such as soups and stews. It is recommended that individuals embrace rest and reflection, and engage in indoor activities that promote relaxation and rejuvenation.

### Daily Self-Care Routines Using Herbal Remedies

The incorporation of herbal remedies into one's daily routine has been demonstrated to support health and well-being. The following section presents a series of suggestions for morning, afternoon, and evening routines.

- *Morning*:

Herbal Tea: Start your day with a cup of energizing herbal tea, such as green tea with ginseng and ginger, to awaken your senses and boost your energy.

Mindfulness Practice: Spend a few minutes in mindfulness or meditation, perhaps using aromatherapy with essential oils like peppermint or rosemary.

- *Afternoon*:

Herbal Snack: Enjoy a snack that includes herbs, such as a smoothie with spirulina or chia seeds infused with lemon balm.

Movement Break: Take a break to stretch or practice yoga, incorporating breathing exercises that include essential oils like eucalyptus to invigorate your senses.

- *Evening*:

Relaxing Bath: End your day with a relaxing herbal bath using lavender and chamomile. This can help soothe your mind and prepare your body for restful sleep.

Sleep Tonic: Drink a calming sleep tonic made with valerian root, passionflower, and lemon balm to promote restful sleep.

## Nourishment Beyond Nutrition

True nourishment is not limited to the physical body; it encompasses mental, emotional, and spiritual well-being as well. Holistic nourishment encompasses the nurturing of all aspects of the individual.

- Mental Nourishment: Engage in activities that stimulate and challenge your mind, such as reading, puzzles, or learning new skills.

- Emotional Nourishment: Practice gratitude and engage in activities that bring joy and fulfillment. Surround yourself with positive relationships and support systems.

- Spiritual Nourishment: Engage in practices that connect you with your deeper self and the world around you, such as meditation, prayer, or spending time in nature.

## Incorporating Movement and Exercise into a Holistic Lifestyle

It is of paramount importance to engage in physical activity on a regular basis in order to maintain optimal health and well-being. It is recommended that individuals integrate movement into their daily routines in a manner that is both natural and enjoyable.

- Daily Exercise: Aim for at least 30 minutes of moderate exercise each day. This could include walking, cycling, dancing, or yoga.

- Mindful Movement: Practice forms of exercise that combine physical movement with mindfulness, such as tai chi, qigong, or yoga. These practices can enhance both physical and mental health.

- Outdoor Activities: Engage in outdoor activities to benefit from fresh air and natural surroundings. Hiking, gardening, and outdoor sports are great ways to stay active and connected to nature.

## *Building a Deeper Connection with Nature*

A robust connection with nature has been demonstrated to have a profound impact on one's health and well-being. The benefits of nature extend beyond the physical realm, offering mental and spiritual rejuvenation.

- Spending Time Outdoors: Make a habit of spending time outdoors daily, whether it's walking in a park, gardening, or simply sitting outside and observing nature.

- Nature Meditation: Practice meditation or mindfulness in natural settings. Focus on the sights, sounds, and smells of the natural world to deepen your sense of connection.

- Eco-Friendly Practices: Adopt sustainable and eco-friendly practices in your daily life. This not only benefits the environment but also fosters a sense of stewardship and connection to the earth.

In Chapter 8, the reader will be guided through the process of managing life's transitions using natural remedies and holistic practices. This chapter will examine the purification of the body and mind through natural means, including the use of simple and effective herbal formulations. It will also explore the integration of natural remedies into contemporary health practices and the transmission of traditional practices to ensure their continued relevance. An understanding of the processes involved in navigating transitions in a healthy and mindful manner allows for the maintenance of equilibrium and well-being during periods of change.

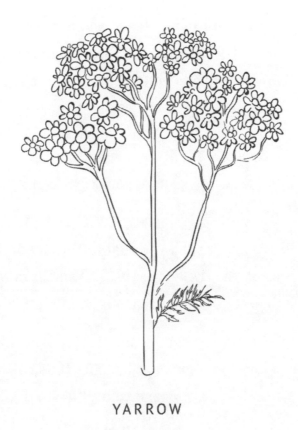

YARROW

# Chapter 8: Managing Transitions

Life is replete with transitions, whether they be seasonal changes, life stage shifts, or periods of personal transformation. The incorporation of natural remedies and holistic practices can assist in maintaining equilibrium and fostering well-being during these transitions. This chapter will examine the potential of natural remedies to purify the body and mind, integrate them into contemporary health practices, and preserve and transmit traditional herbal knowledge.

## Purifying Body and Mind through Natural Means

It is of the utmost importance to engage in detoxifying and purifying practices to maintain health and balance during transitions. Herbal formulations, which are simple and effective, can facilitate this process.

### Simple and Effective Herbal Formulations

The process of detoxification is beneficial in several ways. It helps to eliminate toxins from the body, improve digestion, boost energy levels, and enhance overall well-being. The following recipes are designed to facilitate detoxification and purification:

### 181. *Liver Detox Tea:*

Ingredients: Dandelion root, milk thistle, and burdock root.

Benefits: Dandelion root has been demonstrated to support liver function, while milk thistle has been shown to protect and regenerate liver cells. Burdock root, meanwhile, has been found to aid in overall detoxification.

Recipe: Combine equal parts of dried dandelion root, milk thistle seeds, and burdock root. Steep 1 tablespoon of the blend in 2 cups of hot water for 15 minutes. Strain and drink 1-2 cups daily for a week.

### 182. *Cleansing Green Smoothie:*

Ingredients: Kale, cucumber, apple, lemon, and ginger.

Benefits: Kale provides essential nutrients, cucumber hydrates and flushes out toxins, apple adds fiber, lemon supports digestion, and ginger reduces inflammation.

Recipe: A blend of one cup of chopped kale, one-half cucumber, one apple (cored), the juice of one lemon, and a small piece of fresh ginger with one cup of water is recommended. Drink this smoothie daily in the morning.

### 183. *Detox Bath Soak:*

Ingredients: Epsom salts, baking soda, and lavender essential oil.

Benefits: Epsom salts draw out toxins and relax muscles, baking soda balances pH levels, and lavender essential oil promotes relaxation.

Recipe: Mix 2 cups of Epsom salts, 1 cup of baking soda, and 10 drops of lavender essential oil. The mixture should be added to a warm bath and allowed to soak for a period of 20 to 30 minutes.

## Embracing Natural Remedies in Modern Health Practices

The incorporation of natural remedies into contemporary health regimens can facilitate enhanced overall well-being and provide supplementary assistance during transitions.

Daily Herbal Supplements: It is recommended that herbal supplements be incorporated into one's daily routine in order to support specific health needs. For instance, one might consider taking turmeric capsules to address inflammation or ashwagandha to manage stress.

Holistic Practices: It is recommended that herbal remedies be combined with other holistic practices such as yoga, meditation, and acupuncture in order to create a comprehensive approach to health.

Regular Detox Programs: It is recommended that seasonal detox programs be implemented using herbal teas, dietary changes, and supportive therapies such as massages or saunas in order to maintain optimal health.

## Passing Down Traditions and Ensuring Their Legacy

It is of paramount importance to preserve and transmit herbal traditions in order to ensure the continued survival of this invaluable body of knowledge and to guarantee its benefits to future generations.

Documenting Recipes and Practices: It is recommended that traditional recipes and practices be recorded, along with the associated stories and cultural significance. It is recommended that a family herbal journal or digital archive be created.

Teaching and Sharing: It is of great importance to educate younger generations and the wider community about herbal traditions. One may choose to host workshops, create online content, or simply share one's knowledge with family and friends.

Community Engagement: It is recommended that individuals participate in or support local herbalist groups, community gardens, and herbal education programs. This will foster a community of shared knowledge and practice.

In Chapter 9, we will examine the use of herbal remedies for specific health conditions. This chapter will provide detailed descriptions and usage instructions for a variety of common ailments, including acne, anxiety, arthritis, and asthma. By focusing on targeted herbal treatments, it is possible to effectively manage and alleviate specific health issues with natural remedies. This comprehensive guide will enable the reader to address common health concerns with confidence and in a natural manner.

# Chapter 9: Herbal Remedies for Specific Conditions

Herbal remedies offer effective and natural solutions for a variety of common health conditions. This chapter provides detailed descriptions and usage instructions for specific ailments, thereby empowering the reader to manage and alleviate health issues using the power of nature. This chapter provides an overview of herbal remedies for a range of conditions, including acne, anxiety, arthritis, asthma, and others.

## Remedies for Common Conditions

### Acne

Acne is a persistent and frustrating skin condition. Herbal remedies have been demonstrated to possess anti-inflammatory, antibacterial, and healing properties.

### 184. Tea Tree Oil Spot Treatment:

Ingredients: Tea tree oil.

Benefits: Tea tree oil has antibacterial and anti-inflammatory properties.

Usage: A small quantity of tea tree oil should be applied directly to blemishes using a cotton swab. The recommended dosage is one application per day.

### 185. Calendula Toner:

Ingredients: Calendula flowers, witch hazel.

Benefits: Calendula has been demonstrated to promote healing and reduce inflammation, while witch hazel has been shown to tone and tighten the skin.

Recipe: Steep 1 tablespoon of dried calendula flowers in 1 cup of hot water for 15 minutes. Strain and mix with 1/2 cup of witch hazel. Apply to the face with a cotton pad twice daily.

### Anxiety

Herbal remedies have been demonstrated to have a calming effect on the nervous system, which can result in a reduction in feelings of anxiety.

### 186. Chamomile Tea:

Ingredients: Chamomile flowers.

Benefits: Chamomile is known for its calming and anti-anxiety properties.

Usage: One tablespoon of dried chamomile flowers should be steeped in one cup of hot water for ten minutes. The resulting liquid should be strained and consumed in quantities of one to two cups per day.

### 187. Lavender Essential Oil Inhalation:

Ingredients: Lavender essential oil.

Benefits: Lavender has been demonstrated to promote relaxation and to reduce anxiety.

Usage: Add a few drops of lavender essential oil to a diffuser or inhale directly from the bottle when feeling anxious.

## *Arthritis*

Herbal remedies have been demonstrated to reduce inflammation and pain associated with arthritis.

## *188. Turmeric and Ginger Tea:*

Ingredients: Turmeric root, ginger root, black pepper.

Benefits: Turmeric and ginger have powerful anti-inflammatory properties, and black pepper enhances the absorption of curcumin from turmeric.

Recipe: A solution of 1 teaspoon of turmeric root, 1 teaspoon of ginger root, and a pinch of black pepper in 2 cups of water should be prepared. Simmer for 10 minutes, strain, and drink twice daily.

## *189. Arnica Salve:*

Ingredients: Arnica flowers, coconut oil, beeswax.

Benefits: Arnica reduces pain and inflammation.

Recipe: Infuse 1 cup of coconut oil with 1/2 cup of dried arnica flowers for 2 weeks. The mixture should be strained and heated gently with 1/4 cup of beeswax until the wax has melted. The solution should then be poured into containers and applied to the affected areas as required.

## *Asthma*

Herbal remedies have been demonstrated to be effective in the management of asthma symptoms. They have the potential to support respiratory health and to reduce inflammation.

### *190. Mullein Tea:*

Ingredients: Mullein leaves.

Benefits: Mullein soothes the respiratory tract and reduces inflammation.

Usage: One tablespoon of dried mullein leaves should be steeped in one cup of hot water for a period of 15 minutes. The solution should be strained and consumed twice daily.

### *191. Thyme Steam Inhalation:*

Ingredients: Thyme leaves, hot water.

Benefits: Thyme has been demonstrated to possess antimicrobial and expectorant properties, which collectively facilitate the clearance of respiratory passages..

Usage: Add a handful of dried thyme leaves to a bowl of hot water. Cover your head with a towel and inhale the steam for 5-10 minutes.

## Eczema

Herbal remedies can soothe the skin and reduce inflammation associated with eczema.

### 192. Oatmeal Bath:

Ingredients: Oatmeal, chamomile flowers.

Benefits: Oatmeal soothes and moisturizes the skin, while chamomile reduces inflammation.

Recipe: One cup of oatmeal and one-half cup of dried chamomile flowers should be ground into a fine powder. The mixture should then be added to a warm bath and the subject should remain in the bath for a period of 20 minutes.

### 193. Calendula Cream:

Ingredients: Calendula flowers, coconut oil, beeswax.

Benefits: Calendula has been demonstrated to promote healing and to reduce inflammation.

Recipe: Infuse 1 cup of coconut oil with 1/2 cup of dried calendula flowers for 2 weeks. Strain and heat gently with 1/4 cup of beeswax until melted. Pour into containers and apply to affected areas as needed.

## Insomnia

Herbal remedies can help promote relaxation and improve sleep quality.

### 194. Valerian Root Tea:

Ingredients: Valerian root.

Benefits: Valerian root is renowned for its sedative properties.

Usage: Steep 1 teaspoon of dried valerian root in 1 cup of hot water for 15 minutes. Strain and drink 30 minutes before bedtime.

### 195. Passionflower Tincture:

Ingredients: Passionflower, alcohol (vodka or brandy).

Benefits: Passionflower helps calm the mind and promote sleep.

Recipe: The jar should be filled to one-third of its capacity with dried passionflower. The jar should then be covered with alcohol in order to fill it. Seal and store in a dark place for 4-6 weeks, shaking occasionally. Strain and take 1 teaspoon 30 minutes before bedtime.

## Migraines

Herbal remedies can help reduce the frequency and severity of migraines.

### 196. Feverfew Tea:

Ingredients: Feverfew leaves.

Benefits: Feverfew reduces the frequency and severity of migraines.

Usage: One teaspoon of dried feverfew leaves should be steeped in one cup of hot water for ten minutes. The solution should be strained and consumed on a daily basis.

### 197. Peppermint Oil Rub:

Ingredients: Peppermint essential oil, carrier oil (such as coconut or jojoba oil).

Benefits: Peppermint oil has been demonstrated to relieve headache pain and tension.

Usage: Dilute a few drops of peppermint essential oil in a carrier oil and massage onto the temples and back of the neck.

In Chapter 10, we will examine a range of herbal recipes that have the potential to enhance beauty and vitality. This chapter will examine herbal teas, tinctures, salves, and creams, with a focus on recipes that promote overall health, radiant skin, and vibrant energy. With comprehensive instructions for preparation and utilization, these recipes will assist users in harnessing the potential of herbs to transform their daily wellness routines and achieve a heightened sense of well-being.

# Chapter 10: Transformative Recipes

This chapter explores the world of herbal teas, tinctures, salves, and creams, offering recipes designed to enhance beauty and vitality. These recipes employ the healing properties of herbs to promote overall health, radiant skin, and vibrant energy. With comprehensive instructions for preparation and utilization, these transformative remedies can be integrated into one's daily wellness regimen.

## Herbal Teas, Tinctures, Salves, and Creams

### 198. Radiant Skin Herbal Tea

Ingredients: Rose petals, calendula, nettle, and dandelion root.

Benefits: The use of rose petals and calendula is beneficial for promoting skin health and healing. Nettle provides essential nutrients, while dandelion root supports detoxification.

Recipe: Combine equal parts of dried rose petals, calendula flowers, nettle leaves, and dandelion root. Steep 1 tablespoon of the blend in 2 cups of hot water for 10 minutes. Strain and drink daily.

### 199. Energy Boosting Tincture

Ingredients: Ginseng, ashwagandha, and schisandra berries.

Benefits: Ginseng and ashwagandha boost energy levels and reduce stress, while schisandra berries enhance vitality and endurance.

Recipe: The jar should be filled to one-third of its capacity with a combination of dried ginseng root, ashwagandha root, and schisandra berries. Cover with alcohol (vodka or brandy) to fill the jar. Seal and store in a dark place for 4-6 weeks, shaking occasionally. Strain and take 1 teaspoon twice daily.

## 200. Rejuvenating Face Cream

Ingredients: Aloe vera gel, rosehip oil, lavender essential oil, and beeswax.

Benefits: Aloe vera soothes and hydrates, rosehip oil provides antioxidants and promotes skin regeneration, lavender essential oil calms and heals, and beeswax forms a protective barrier.

Recipe: Melt 1/4 cup of beeswax in a double boiler. Once the mixture has reached a temperature that is no longer conducive to further heating, 1/2 cup of aloe vera gel, 1/4 cup of rosehip oil, and 10 drops of lavender essential oil should be added. The mixture should be whisked until it is well combined, after which it should be poured into a jar. This product should be applied daily as a moisturizer.

## 201. Detoxifying Body Scrub

Ingredients: Sea salt, coconut oil, lemon zest, and rosemary essential oil.

Benefits: The application of sea salt exfoliates and detoxifies the skin, while the use of coconut oil moisturizes. The addition of lemon zest provides vitamin C, and the incorporation of rosemary essential oil stimulates circulation.

Recipe: Mix 1 cup of sea salt with 1/2 cup of melted coconut oil, the zest of one lemon, and 10 drops of rosemary essential oil. Store in a jar and use as a body scrub in the shower.

## 202. Hair Strengthening Rinse

Ingredients: Rosemary, nettle, and apple cider vinegar.

Benefits: Rosemary stimulates hair growth, nettle strengthens hair and reduces dandruff, and apple cider vinegar balances scalp pH.

Recipe: One-quarter cup of each of the dried rosemary and nettle is to be steeped in two cups of boiling water for a period of 30 minutes. Strain and mix with 1/2 cup of apple cider vinegar. Use as a final rinse after shampooing.

## 203. Anti-Aging Herbal Serum

Ingredients: Frankincense essential oil, jojoba oil, and vitamin E oil.

Benefits: Frankincense essential oil reduces wrinkles and promotes skin regeneration, jojoba oil moisturizes, and vitamin E oil provides antioxidants.

Recipe: Mix 2 tablespoons of jojoba oil with 10 drops of frankincense essential oil and 1 teaspoon of vitamin E oil. It is recommended that the product be stored in a dropper bottle and that a few drops be applied to the face and neck on a daily basis.

## 204. Soothing Eye Cream

Ingredients: Chamomile, cucumber, and shea butter.

Benefits: Chamomile reduces puffiness and inflammation, cucumber hydrates and soothes, and shea butter moisturizes.

Recipe: One-quarter cup of shea butter should be infused with two tablespoons of dried chamomile flowers and two tablespoons of cucumber juice. The shea butter should be melted and then the chamomile and cucumber should be added. The mixture should then be strained and poured into a small jar. The application of the aforementioned mixture should be conducted around the eyes prior to bedtime.

## 205. Herbal Lip Balm

Ingredients: Beeswax, coconut oil, honey, and peppermint essential oil.

Benefits: The protective and sealing properties of beeswax, the moisturising effects of coconut oil, the healing properties of honey, and the refreshing tingle provided by peppermint essential oil are all beneficial to the skin.

Recipe: Melt 1 tablespoon of beeswax with 1 tablespoon of coconut oil and 1 teaspoon of honey. Remove from heat and add 5 drops of peppermint essential oil. Pour into lip balm tubes or small containers and let cool.

## 206. Vitality Boosting Green Smoothie

Ingredients: Spinach, kale, banana, avocado, chia seeds, and spirulina.

Benefits: Spinach and kale provide essential nutrients, banana and avocado add creaminess and healthy fats, chia seeds offer fiber and omega-3s, and spirulina boosts energy and detoxifies.

Recipe: The preparation of a nutritional beverage begins with the blending of one cup of spinach, one cup of kale, one banana, one-half avocado, one tablespoon of chia seeds, and one teaspoon of spirulina with one to two cups of water or almond milk. This beverage may be consumed as a breakfast or snack.

## 207. Anti-Inflammatory Turmeric Latte

Ingredients: Turmeric, ginger, cinnamon, coconut milk, and honey.

Benefits: The incorporation of turmeric and ginger into a recipe can serve to reduce inflammation. The addition of cinnamon can provide antioxidants, while coconut milk can provide healthy fats. Finally, honey can be used to sweeten and soothe a recipe.

Recipe: Mix 1 teaspoon of turmeric powder, 1/2 teaspoon of ginger powder, 1/2 teaspoon of cinnamon powder, and 1 tablespoon of honey with 2 cups of warm coconut milk. Whisk until well combined and drink as a soothing beverage.

## 208. Herbal Sleep Pillow Spray

Ingredients: Lavender essential oil, chamomile essential oil, and distilled water.

Benefits: Lavender and chamomile promote relaxation and improve sleep quality.

Recipe: The mixture of 20 drops of lavender essential oil, 20 drops of chamomile essential oil, and 1/2 cup of distilled water in a spray bottle is to be prepared.. Shake well and spray onto your pillow before bedtime.

## 209. Glowing Skin Face Mask

Ingredients: Honey, oatmeal, and rose water.

Benefits: Honey moisturizes and heals, oatmeal exfoliates and soothes, and rose water tones and hydrates.

Recipe: Mix 2 tablespoons of honey, 1 tablespoon of finely ground oatmeal, and 1 tablespoon of rose water into a paste. The application of the product to the face should be followed by a 15-20 minute period of retention before rinsing with warm water.

## 210. Invigorating Herbal Bath Salts

Ingredients: Epsom salts, dried rosemary, dried mint, and eucalyptus essential oil.

Benefits: Epsom salts relax muscles and detoxify, rosemary and mint invigorate, and eucalyptus essential oil clears the sinuses.

Recipe: Two cups of Epsom salts should be combined with one-quarter cup of each of dried rosemary and dried mint. Finally, add 10 drops of eucalyptus essential oil. The mixture should be stored in a jar and added to a warm bath at a concentration of approximately half a cup.

## 211. Anti-Stress Herbal Tincture

Ingredients: Ashwagandha, holy basil, and alcohol (vodka or brandy).

Benefits: Ashwagandha and holy basil are adaptogens that assist in the management of stress and the promotion of relaxation.

Recipe: Fill a jar one-third full with dried ashwagandha root and holy basil leaves. Cover with alcohol to fill the jar. Seal and store in a dark place for 4-6 weeks, shaking occasionally. Strain and take 1 teaspoon twice daily.

## 212. Radiant Hair Oil

Ingredients: Coconut oil, argan oil, and rosemary essential oil.

Benefits: Coconut oil moisturizes and protects, argan oil adds shine and reduces frizz, and rosemary essential oil stimulates hair growth.

Recipe: A solution of 1/4 cup of coconut oil, 1/4 cup of argan oil, and 10 drops of rosemary essential oil should be prepared by mixing the ingredients together. Store in a bottle and apply a small amount to the hair, focusing on the ends.

## 213. Herbal Foot Soak

Ingredients: Epsom salts, baking soda, lavender essential oil, and dried chamomile flowers.

Benefits: Epsom salts relax muscles, baking soda softens the skin, lavender essential oil calms, and chamomile soothes.

Recipe: Mix 1 cup of Epsom salts with 1/4 cup of baking soda, 10 drops of lavender essential oil, and 1/4 cup of dried chamomile flowers. The feet should be immersed in a basin of warm water for a period of 20 to 30 minutes.

## 214. Uplifting Citrus Body Lotion

Ingredients: Shea butter, coconut oil, orange essential oil, and lemon essential oil.

Benefits: Shea butter and coconut oil deeply moisturize, while orange and lemon essential oils uplift and refresh.

Recipe: The shea butter and coconut oil should be combined in a heat-resistant container and melted together at a temperature that does not exceed

120 degrees Celsius. Once the mixture has cooled to a temperature below 100 degrees Celsius, 10 drops of each orange and lemon essential oil should be added. The mixture should be whisked until it is well combined, after which it should be poured into a jar. The lotion should be applied daily to the body.

### 215. Clarifying Herbal Face Steam

Ingredients: Chamomile, peppermint, and rosemary.

Benefits: Chamomile has a soothing effect, peppermint provides a refreshing sensation, and rosemary has a clarifying effect.

Recipe: Add a handful of dried chamomile flowers, peppermint leaves, and rosemary leaves to a bowl of hot water. Lean over the bowl with a towel over your head and steam your face for 5-10 minutes.

### 216. Joint Soothing Salve

Ingredients: Arnica, cayenne, ginger, and beeswax.

Benefits: Arnica reduces inflammation, cayenne and ginger improve circulation, and beeswax forms a protective barrier.

Recipe: One cup of olive oil should be infused with 1/2 cup of dried arnica flowers, 1/4 cup of dried cayenne pepper, and 1/4 cup of dried ginger for a period of two weeks. Strain and heat gently with 1/4 cup of beeswax until melted. Pour into containers and apply to sore joints as needed.

## 217. Refreshing Facial Toner

Ingredients: Witch hazel, cucumber juice, and rose water.

Benefits: Witch hazel tones and tightens, cucumber hydrates, and rose water soothes and balances.

Recipe: Mix 1/2 cup of witch hazel, 1/4 cup of cucumber juice, and 1/4 cup of rose water. The product should be stored in a sealed bottle and applied to the face with a cotton pad following cleansing.

# Illustrations of the main herbs used

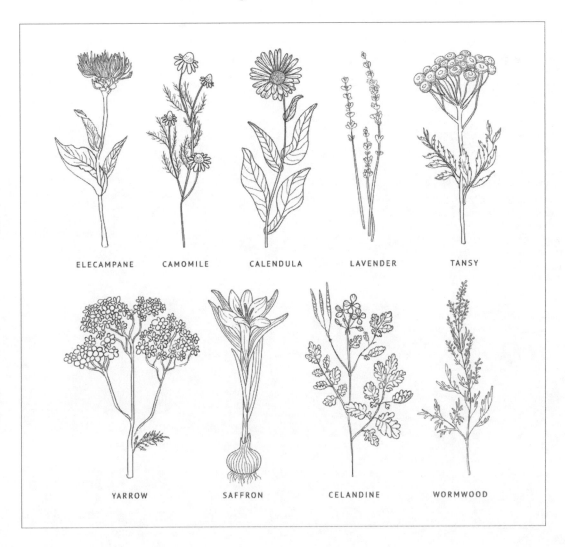

ELECAMPANE    CAMOMILE    CALENDULA    LAVENDER    TANSY

YARROW    SAFFRON    CELANDINE    WORMWOOD

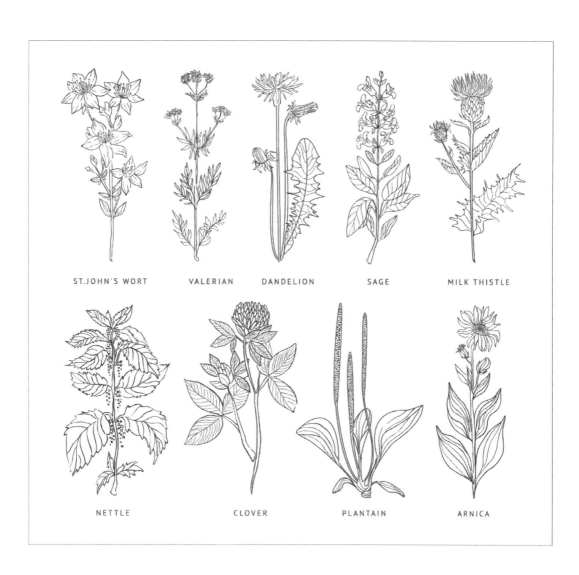

ST.JOHN'S WORT      VALERIAN      DANDELION      SAGE      MILK THISTLE

NETTLE      CLOVER      PLANTAIN      ARNICA

# Conclusion

As we conclude our examination of the vast and multifaceted realm of herbal remedies and holistic health practices, it is essential to contemplate the journey we have traversed and to anticipate the limitless potential that lies ahead. This book has provided you with a foundation, a starting point from which to explore and deepen your understanding of natural healing. Nevertheless, the process of acquiring knowledge and understanding is an ongoing and ever-evolving endeavor, with boundless potential for growth and fulfillment.

## Encouraging Continued Learning and Exploration

One of the most appealing aspects of natural healing is its capacity for continuous evolution. New discoveries and insights are continually being made, driven by a synthesis of traditional wisdom and modern science. As you continue on your path, it is recommended that you remain curious. It is recommended that you embrace the desire to learn more about the plants and practices that can enhance your well-being. It is recommended that you explore new topics, experiment with different remedies, and observe how your body responds. The field of natural healing is as expansive and diverse as the natural world itself, offering limitless potential for growth and discovery.

It is important to note that the most profound learning often occurs through personal experience. While books, courses, and mentors are invaluable resources, one's own observations and experiences will deepen one's understanding in unique and meaningful ways. It is important to pay close attention to how different remedies affect you, taking notes and refining your practices based on what you discover. This personalized approach to learning not only enhances one's knowledge but also strengthens one's connection to one's own body and its needs.

## *Embracing Nature as a Constant in Health and Wellness*

This book has consistently underscored the profound connection between nature and health. The concept of nature as a mere backdrop to our lives is a narrow and incomplete one. Rather, nature is an integral part of our existence, a source of endless healing and wellness. From the air we breathe to the food we eat and the remedies we use, nature provides us with all the resources we require to maintain and restore our health.

The concept of embracing nature is not merely limited to the utilization of herbal remedies; rather, it encompasses the cultivation of a lifestyle that honors and integrates natural rhythms and cycles. It is recommended that individuals spend time outdoors, observe the changing seasons, and align their daily activities with the natural world. This connection fosters a sense of balance, harmony, and well-being that is essential for the maintenance of true health.

As you continue your journey, it is important to remember that nature is a constant and ever-present source of support and inspiration. Whether one is confronting health challenges or merely striving to maintain a state of well-being, turning to nature will consistently offer guidance and healing. The flora, fauna, and natural cycles are allies that are ready to assist in the nurturing of the body, mind, and spirit.

## A Call to Action

As this book draws to a close, I urge you to apply the knowledge you have acquired to your daily life. It is advisable to commence with minor alterations and subsequently to build upon them in a gradual manner. It is recommended that you create your own herbal remedies, establish daily routines that align with your natural rhythms, and continue to engage in learning and growth. It is recommended that you share your knowledge and experiences with others, thus fostering a community of like-minded individuals who value and practice natural healing.

Above all, maintain a state of curiosity and an open mind. The field of herbal remedies and holistic health is vast and full of unexpected discoveries. There is always more to learn, more to explore, and more to discover. It is recommended that the journey be one of continuous growth, guided by the wisdom of nature and the knowledge that the individual has the power to heal and nurture themselves.

In conclusion, it is my hope that this book has inspired you to embrace the beauty and efficacy of natural healing. It is my hope that you will find joy, health, and fulfillment in the practices you adopt and the discoveries you make. It is important to remember that nature is always available to provide an endless bounty of resources and unwavering support. It is recommended that you embrace this knowledge, learn from it, and allow it to guide you on your journey to optimal health and wellness.